A Practical Guide to Health Assessment

A Practical Guide to Health Assessment

Marilyn Shelley Leasia, RN, MSN, FNP
Chief Nurse Practitioner
Department of Medicine, Attending Oriented Service
Montefiore Medical Center
Bronx, New York

Frances Donovan Monahan, PhD, RN
Professor and Chair
Department of Nursing
Rockland Community College
Suffern, New York

W.B. SAUNDERS COMPANY
A Division of Harcourt Brace & Company
Philadelphia   London   Toronto   Montreal   Sydney   Tokyo

W.B. SAUNDERS COMPANY
A Division of Harcourt Brace & Company

The Curtis Center
Independence Square West
Philadelphia, Pennsylvania 19106

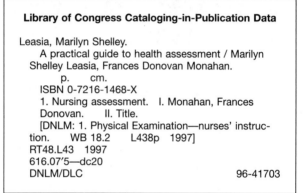

Library of Congress Cataloging-in-Publication Data

Leasia, Marilyn Shelley.
　A practical guide to health assessment / Marilyn
Shelley Leasia, Frances Donovan Monahan.
　　　　p.　　cm.
　ISBN 0-7216-1468-X
　1. Nursing assessment.　I. Monahan, Frances
Donovan.　　II. Title.
　[DNLM: 1. Physical Examination—nurses' instruc-
tion.　　WB 18.2　　L438p　1997]
RT48.L43　1997
616.07′5—dc20
DNLM/DLC　　　　　　　　　　　　　　96-41703

A PRACTICAL GUIDE TO HEALTH ASSESSMENT
　　　　　　　　　　　　　　　ISBN 0-7216-1468-X

Printed in the United States of America.

Last digit is the print number:　9　8　7　6　5　4　3　2　1

Dedication

For my brother Michael, who humbles us by reminding us of our painful limitations.

For my niece Jessica, who encourages us on by showing we are capable of extraordinary triumphs.

MARILYN SHELLEY LEASIA

Dedicated with all my love to my husband William T. Monahan, my son Michael McCain Monahan, my daughter Kerryane Torpey Monahan, and my aunt Claire T. Torpey.

FRANCES D. MONAHAN

CONTRIBUTORS LIST

Sue-Ann Eitches, MA, RN, (BSN)
Associate Professor
Department of Nursing
Rockland Community College
Suffern, New York

Ellen M. Flynn, JD, MSN, CPNP
Clinical Preceptor
Hunter College
Hunter-Bellevue School of Nursing
Columbia University School of Nursing
New York, New York
Pediatric Nurse Practitioner
Gergely Pediatrics
Garrison, New York

Janet Drew Reynolds, MSN
Assistant Professor
Seton Hall University
College of Nursing
South Orange, New Jersey

Joan Stackhouse
Associate Professor, retired
Rockland Community College
Suffern, New York

Acknowledgments

T he authors wish to thank Barbara Nelson Cullen, Senior Editor, Marie Pelcin, Editorial Assistant, and Pat Morrison, Art and Design Director of W. B. Saunders Company; the staff of Dartmouth Publishing Inc. for their excellent preparation of the artwork for the book; and to Tony Caruso for putting it all together. A special thank you to Sue Anne Eitches, Ellen Flynn, Janet Drew Reynolds, and Joan Stackhouse for their professionalism, cooperation, and attention to deadlines.

No man is an island, and neither, I have learned, are any books! I am so grateful for the assistance of so many people whose professional contributions carried *A Practical Guide to Health Assessment* to its final publication. I would like to give special thanks to my partner and co-editor Frances Donovan Monahan whose experienced advice and special friendship truly made this book a joy to write and to Barbara Nelson Cullen, Senior Editor of Nursing Books at W.B. Saunders for painstakingly guiding us through every step of the publishing process. Special thanks are also due to Janet Drew Reynolds for her Geriatric Considerations and Ellen M. Flynn for her Pediatric Considerations included at the end of each chapter. I would also like to thank a few key people whom I did know as well as the countless others whom I did not know at W.B. Saunders. These include: Marie Pelcin, Editorial Assistant; David Kerprich, Manager; and Lanie Meriwether, Assistant of Nursing Marketing. I would also like to thank our artists at Dartmouth whom I believe had the most difficult job of creating, correcting and recorrecting new and original artwork for the book. I would like to thank Denise Black Gold, Development Editor, for her assistance with the editing of the enormous amount of artwork generated for the book. I would also like to give very special thanks to Tony Caruso who did a magnificent job making a silk purse out of a sow's ear with the actual layout and publishing of the book. And last, but certainly not least, I would like to thank my daughter Dora Sobze, for her help with the tedious jobs of Xeroxing, cutting and pasting; my husband Dr. Isdor Sobze, who patiently provided around the clock assistance with computer and word-processing issues; my wonderful Father, Richard S. Leasia; mothers, Marilyn J. Jacobsen and Florence M. Leasia; and family who have always supported me no matter how unbelievable my endeavors.

REVIEWERS LIST

Louvenia Carter, PhD, RN, CNA
Northwestern State University of Louisiana
Shreveport, Louisiana

Roselyn B. Holloway, RN, MSN
Methodist Hospital School of Nursing
Lubbock, Texas

Denise Marie LeBlanc, RN, BScn
Humber College
Continuing Education Nursing
Toronto, Ontario

Nancy Otterness, RN, MS
Boise State University
Department of Nursing
Boise, Idaho

Deborah Vendittelli, RN, MSN, C, ANP
Schoolcraft College, Livonia, Michigan
Huron Valley Hospital, Commerce, Michigan

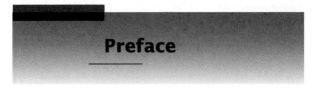

Preface

The rapidly changing health care delivery system has made strong history, taking physical examination skills essential for today's practitioners. However, until now, only large textbooks provided the detailed, heavily illustrated content necessary for learning health assessment.

Our aim with this book is to provide students with a portable guide that is easy to use and provides the detailed information they need to take a client's health history and perform a physical examination. The content is presented in clear step-by-step increments, with the liberal use of illustrations to help reinforce learning. We also include a color plate to illustrate eye and ear abnormalities that cannot be adequately depicted in a line drawing.

Using a body systems approach, each chapter addresses the entire life span by including both pediatric and geriatric considerations. Where appropriate, we have also included racial and cultural content, to address the needs of our diverse client population.

By combining our respective areas of expertise as nurse practitioner and educator, we have worked to reconcile the reality of clinical practice with the needs of today's students. We think you will agree the result is a book that will not only teach the skills of history taking and physical examination, but will leave the reader with a true understanding of the importance of health assessment.

SHELLEY LEASIA
FRANCES D. MONAHAN

Notice

Assessment is an ever-changing field. Standard safety precautions must be followed, but as new research and clinical experience broaden our knowledge, changes in treatment and drug therapy become necessary or appropriate. The editors of this work have carefully checked the generic and trade drug names and verified drug dosages to ensure that the dosage information in this work is accurate and in accord with the standards accepted at the time of publication. Readers are advised, however, to check the product information currently provided by the manufacturer of each drug to be administered to be certain that changes have not been made in the recommended dose or in the contraindications for administration. This is of particular importance in regard to new or infrequently used drugs. It is the responsibility of the treating physician, relying on experience and knowledge of the patient, to determine dosages and the best treatment for the patient. The editors cannot be responsible for misuse or misapplication of the material in this work.

THE PUBLISHER

Contents

PLATE I

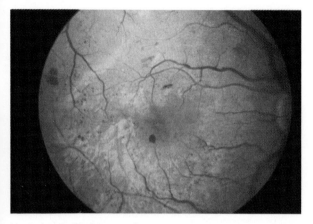

Normal optic fundus

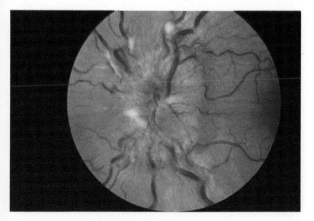

Optic fundus of a client with diabetes

PLATE II

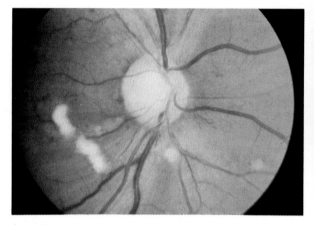

Optic fundus of a client with hypertension

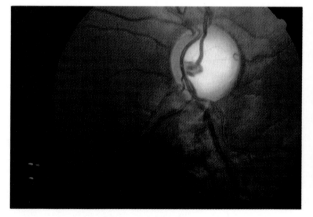

Optic fundus of a client with glaucoma

PLATE III

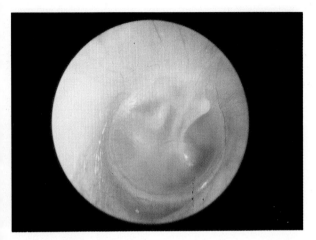

Normal tympanic membrane

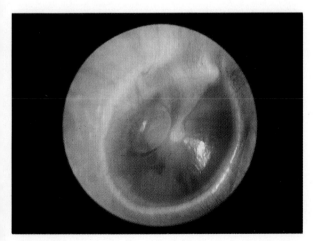

Otitis media

PLATE IV

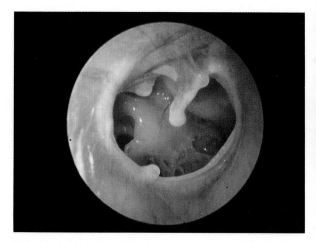

Perforated tympanic membrane

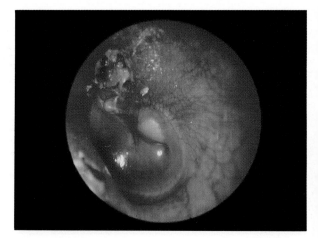

Cholesteatoma

1

The Health History

The health history is a collection of subjective data that includes information on both the patient's past and present health status. It is used in conjunction with the physical examination and laboratory findings as a basis for drawing conclusions about an individual's state of health. It allows positive aspects of health and health habits as well as abnormal symptoms, health problems, health teaching needs, and health concerns to be identified.

COMPONENTS OF A COMPREHENSIVE HEALTH HISTORY

Date history obtained
Source of history (patient, spouse, relative, friend, medical records, etc.)
Interpreter if used (name, role, or relationship to patient)
Reason for seeking health care (e.g., routine physical examination, referral by another health care provider, presence of signs or symptoms of illness); record in patient's own words

Patient Profile Data

Name
Address
Telephone number

Social Security number
Date of birth (day, month, year)
Place of birth (city, state, country)
Sex
Race/ethnic origin
Marital status (single, married, divorced, widowed)
Religious preference (religion as well as name of house of
  worship, spiritual advisor if appropriate)
Education
Occupation
Hobbies
Military service
Name of physician
Source of referral
Insurance information (Medicare/Medicaid number, other
  insurance name and number)

Present Illness Data

Date of onset
Symptoms (type, location, frequency, duration)
Precipitating and/or associated factors
Relieving and alleviating factors (e.g., timing, setting)
Effect on other body functions
Effect on ADLs and life-style
Treatment measures utilized (type and frequency)
Effectiveness of treatment measures

Present Health Status (Apart from Present Illness)

Perceived state of health apart from current illness (patient's perception of self as healthy, prone to specific ail-
  ments, always having some health problem, etc.)
Existing health problems apart from the present illness
  (type, management)
Physical handicaps (type, management)
Prescription medications currently taken (name, dose,
  route, frequency, for how long, by whom prescribed, reason for taking, side effects)
OTC medications (name, dose, frequency, reason for taking, effectiveness)

(Also question regarding use of borrowed drugs. Be sure
to warn of the dangers of this practice after asking; do
not warn prior to asking as it could make the patient
hesitant to admit to their use.)

Home remedies used (type, frequency, reason for use, effectiveness)

Allergies (food, drug, environmental; type of reaction,
management)

Immunization status (dates and types, e.g.,
measles/mumps/rubella, polio, pertussis/tetanus, tetanus
booster, influenza, diphtheria, hepatitis; Table 1–1)

Past Personal Health Data

Childhood illnesses (e.g., strep throat, scarlet fever, rheu-
matic fever, polio, measles, mumps, rubella, chicken pox)

Serious adult illnesses (e.g., diabetes, hypertension, heart
disease, cancer; treatment)

Accidents/injuries (type, date, treatment, sequelae)

Hospitalizations (date, cause, hospital, physician, treatment, length of stay)

Surgery (date, type, postoperative course, name of hospital
and surgeon)

Obstetric history (number of pregnancies, viable deliveries;
course of completed pregnancies, type of labor and
delivery; sex, weight, and general condition of each
neonate; postpartum course; number of spontaneous abortions, number of therapeutic abortions, age of pregnancy
at time of each abortion)

Exposure to toxins or environmental pollutants (type,
amount of exposure, untoward effects)

Blood transfusions (dates, number, untoward effects)

Family Medical Data

Age and health, or age and cause of death of parents,
grandparents, siblings

Blood relative history of heart disease, hypertension, cere-
brovascular disease, diabetes, anemia, cancer, arthritis,
alcoholism, obesity, tuberculosis, renal disorders, seizure
disorders, or mental illness (specific disease, age of onset,
management)

T A B L E   I–I
Standard Schedule of Immunizations

Age	Immunization(s)	Abbreviation
Birth	Hepatitis B virus vaccine	HBV-1
2 months	Diphtheria toxoid, tetanus toxoid, pertussis vaccine	DTP-1
	Oral poliovirus vaccine, live	OPV-1
	Hemophilus influenzae type B-diphtheria CRM197 protein conjugate	HbOC
	Hepatitis B virus vaccine	HBV-2
4 months	Diphtheria toxoid, tetanus toxoid, pertussis vaccine	DTP-2
	Oral poliovirus vaccine	OPV-2
	Hemophilus influenzae type B-diphtheria CRM197 protein conjugate	HbOC
6 months	Diphtheria toxoid, tetanus toxoid, pertussis vaccine	DTP-3
	Hemophilus influenzae type B-diphtheria CRM197 protein conjugate	HbOC
	Hepatitis B virus vaccine	HBV-3
15 months	Measles, mumps, rubella virus vaccine, live	MMR-1
	Diphtheria toxoid, tetanus toxoid, pertussis vaccine	DTP-4
	Oral poliovirus vaccine	OPV-3
	Hemophilus influenzae type B-diphtheria CRM197 protein conjugate	HbOC
4–6 years	Diphtheria toxoid, tetanus toxoid, pertussis vaccine	DTP-5
	Oral poliovirus vaccine	OPV-4
	Measles, mumps, rubella virus vaccine, live	MMR-2
14–16 years and every 10 years throughout life	Tetanus and diphtheria toxoids (adult types)	Td

Table continued on following page

Communicable disease in close family members, including
spouse and children (type, date of onset, treatment)
Age and health history of spouse and children
Record family history in diagram or genogram form for
easy reference (Fig. 1–1).

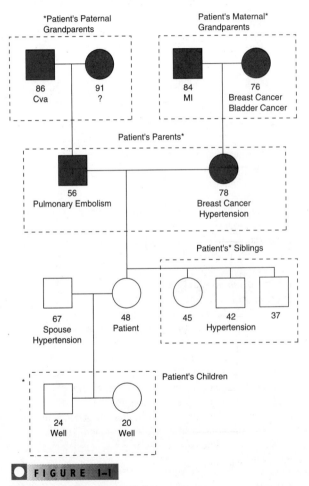

FIGURE 1–1

Family medical history recorded as a genogram.

Life-Style Data

Ability to perform basic ADLs, such as:

- toileting
- bathing
- grooming
- dressing
- walking
- climbing stairs
- eating
- using the telephone
- shopping
- cooking
- housekeeping/cleaning
- laundry
- managing money
- transportation
- taking medications

(Indicate ability as I—*independent;* A—*needs assistance;*
  D—*dependent.*)
Usual daily activities
Work (type, responsibilities, hours, attitude toward,
  stresses/problems)
Perceived role in family unit
Exercise patterns (type, frequency, duration)
Leisure activities/hobbies (type, time involved)
Participation in social groups (type, amount)
Sexual orientation
Sexual activity (frequency, type, use of contraceptives)
Rest/sleep (usual sleep time; quality of sleep; difficulty
  falling alseep, staying asleep, or waking up; sleep aids
  used; sleep routine (e.g., light on, music))
Nutritional intake (time, type and amount of foods and flu-
  ids typically consumed in a 24-hour period, recent
  change in appetite, special diet)
Eating habits
Adequate finances for food
Caffeine intake (source, amount, pattern of use)

Use of alcohol (type, pattern of use, amount used, number of years used, effect of use on work)

Use of tobacco (type, amount per day, number of years used)

Use of illegal drugs (type, pattern of use, amount used, number of years used)

Recent trips to foreign countries (specify)

Health Management Data

Understanding of personal health status

Personal health goals

Routine hygienic practices (type, frequency, cultural taboos)

Date of last physical examination

Health screening tests (e.g., mammogram, Pap smear, stool for occult blood; type, date, results)

Self-examination (e.g., breast, testicular, skin; date of most recent self-examination; frequency; technique)

Date of most recent dental examination

Date of most recent eye examination

Date of most recent hearing examination

Date and results of most recent PPD or chest x-ray

Date and result of most recent ECG

Expectations of health care workers

Psychosocial Data

Perception of self (e.g., strengths, weaknesses, appearance, ability to function)

Sources of personal stress

Ability to cope (coping mechanisms used in the past, methods of relieving stress, persons/things that aid coping)

Perceived effect of feelings about present illness

Significant others (who, relationship to patient, location)

Family relationships (family members, proximity of residence, type of interaction between and among family members, patient's role in the family, how and by whom family decisions are made, how family copes with problems, how family is coping with the patient's illness)

Religious practices desired during illness (e.g., bible
reading; visit from minister, hospital chaplain, medicine
man, faith healer; wearing of medals; wearing of a medicine bag)

Home environment

- Type (e.g., house or apartment, number of rooms,
  owned or rented, one or more stories, number of stairs)
- Facilities in home (e.g., telephone, heat, furnishings in
  good repair)
- Number and age of others in household
- Type of neighborhood (e.g., urban, suburban, or rural;
  traffic; sidewalks; gangs; amount of crime)
- Available transportation (car, bus, walking)
- Access to shopping, house of worship, drug store, health
  care facilities, education facilities
- Type of (elderly, or mix of ages, none during the day,
  working) and relationship to neighbors

History of physical or sexual abuse (dates, type, by whom,
action taken, stage of problem resolution)

Recent changes in life-style

Support system available (note cultural variations (life
ways) that affect support, such as Mexican-American *suc-
corama*)

Review of Systems

See history and current status questions at beginning of
Chapters 3 through 21.

GUIDELINES FOR OBTAINING A HEALTH HISTORY

Greet patient by name using appropriate title (e.g., Mr.,
Mrs., Ms., Reverend, Sister, Doctor).

Introduce yourself, giving your name, title, and role.

Provide a private, quiet environment free of interruptions.

Ensure that the patient is as comfortable as possible prior
to beginning the history (i.e., comfortable room
temperature, comfortable position, empty bladder, good
but not harsh lighting).

Sit at eye level 4 to 5 feet apart from the patient.

(Keep in mind that some patients such as those of traditional Hispanic, East Indian and Middle Eastern background may prefer closer physical proximity and may
negatively perceive an effort on your part to reestablish
distance if they have moved closer to you.)

Avoid sitting with a bright light behind you, which creates
glare and makes it difficult for the patient to look at you
without squinting or shading the eyes.

Be calm, confident yet empathetic, and nonjudgmental.

Explain the purpose of obtaining the health history.

Reassure the patient regarding the confidentiality of the
history.

Use clear, unambiguous language appropriate to the background of the patient. Avoid both use of terms that the
patient may not understand and oversimplification.

Ask one question at a time (e.g., "Are you allergic to
foods?" as opposed to "Are you allergic to foods, drugs,
animal dander, pollen?")

Begin with neutral, factual questions; gradually progress
to questions of a potentially sensitive or embarrassing
nature.

Ask direct closed-ended questions (call for a one- or two-
word answer) to obtain factual information in a time-
efficient manner.

Ask open-ended questions (cannot be answered in one or
two words) to obtain information about perceptions,
understandings, and feelings.

Avoid leading questions (i.e., those that suggest a correct
or acceptable answer). (Keep in mind this is especially
critical with Asian patients, who often place a strong
value on social harmony.)

Allow time for the patient to consider the question, orga-
nize his or her thoughts, and respond fully.

Do not "put words in the patient's mouth"; allow the patient to use his or her own words.

Give the patient your undivided attention and acknowledge
listening by nodding or saying "Uh hum," "yes," or "I
hear you."

Establish eye contact appropriate to the cultural background of the patient. (Keep in mind that some patients, such as traditional Asians, Native Americans, and Arabs, may consider direct eye contact as impolite or aggressive and may keep their own eyes averted or on the floor).

Promote accurate, complete communication by using facilitative verbal responses as described in Table 1–2.

Be alert to nonverbal communication.

Validate your understanding of the patient's verbal and nonverbal communication by stating your understanding of the communication and asking the patient to confirm or deny it.

Take brief notes (key words, phrases, times) during the history; do not rely totally on your memory. Do not write so extensively that rapport between you and the patient is lost.

If the patient is hearing impaired, face him or her when speaking; enunciate clearly; use a low tone of voice; speak to the better ear; and use an amplifying or other assistive device as necessary.

Use a bilingual health team member or trained interpreter as needed with non-English-speaking patients or those for whom English is a second language. Avoid use of relatives or friends as interpreters because of issues of confidentiality and lack of familiarity with medical terms. For maximum accuracy, use line-by-line translation, not summary translation.

Geriatric Considerations

Older patients' histories take longer because they have more information to tell. Multiple interviews may be more productive and less fatiguing for the frail patient. Collect the most important historical data first.

Frail patients may be accompanied by a spouse, adult child, or friend. Determine the patient's wishes regarding the presence of others during the health history.

Conduct the interview in a quiet room with adequate lighting to compensate for sensory deficits.

Older patients' chronic health problems often impact on function. When functions cannot be performed, assess what support services are available to meet the need.

T A B L E 1–2
Facilitative Verbal Responses

Facilitative Response	Behavioral Examples	Theoretical Notes
1. Approach the patient with acceptance and genuine respect.	This is best conveyed by facial expression, tone of voice, posture, and attention to the patient's comfort and time constraints: *"What brings you here?"* *"What would you like to talk about?"* *"Would you like information about ___?"* *"Do you have a plan regarding ___?"* *"What do you think about ___?"* AVOID: *"My advice to you is ___."* *"Let me take care of those problems for you."* *"You shouldn't feel that ___."* *"Being afraid of surgery is silly in this day of high technology."* *"Don't worry! Everything will be fine!"*	Acceptance of the person does not necessarily mean approval of all the behaviors, attitudes, and feelings of the patient. It is crucial to distinguish between the person and the behaviors, which may be totally contrary to your value system. Genuine respect is based on the assumption that each person or situation has potential for change. The integrity and the ability of the patient to make satisfactory decisions about life, given appropriate help, must be respected. This avoids the pitfalls of giving advice, being glib, attempting to rescue the patient, or belittling the patient's feelings. Avoidance of cliches and stereotypes is also basic to respect. Reassurance statements like *"Don't worry!"* do not really reassure. To provide reassurance, be trustworthy and communicate empathy and respect. Also, give correct information at the time the patient needs it.

Table continued on following page

TABLE 1-2
Facilitative Verbal Responses *(Continued)*

Facilitative Response	Behavioral Examples	Theoretical Notes
2. Reflect feelings expressed by the patient verbally and nonverbally.	*"You seem very concerned."* *"I sense that you are annoyed."* *"It must be so frightening."* *"Sounds like you are pretty discouraged."* DO NOT SAY: *"I understand how you feel."* Avoid emotionally charged words until the patient uses them. Say: *"You must feel so alone."* instead of *"You feel abandoned."* AVOID: *"You are enraged* (depressed)." *"What a panic you are in!"* *"You must despise that!"* *"Are you suicidal?"* Instead say: *"Do you ever think of hurting yourself?"*	Reflection of the patient's feelings communicates empathy and builds trust essential to a therapeutic relationship. Reflection seeks to demonstrate understanding of what the patient is experiencing. It is rarely appropriate for a nurse to say, *"I understand how you feel."* Only the patient can say, *"The nurse understands."* Use gentle terms to assess the degree of feelings initially. Once the patient uses a more potent, emotionally charged word, it is appropriate for you to use it. Be aware of cultural and age differences in regard to charged words. For example, elderly American women, often raised to believe that a lady should not get angry, may feel the word "angry" is taboo. Asians may also be uncomfortable with the word "angry," whereas persons under age 50 raised in the culture of the United States, are likely to have no difficulty with it.

3. Encourage expression of feelings, perceptions, and attitudes by using open-ended questions.	*"Tell me about —."* *"What were you feeling (thinking) when that happened?"* *"Describe what that was like."* *"Go on."* Wait attentively during periods of silence to give the patient time to organize his/her thoughts.	Use of open-ended questions to encourage expression allows you to learn what is important to the patient rather than make assumptions based upon your priorities. It also allows the patient to verbalize feelings and perceptions and thus begin to identify the cause of vague inner turmoil and to work on the problem. Even when patients already understand the nature of their problems, the opportunity to ventilate is extremely helpful. "Talking it out" is a major stress reducer. It is also true that persons who "talk it out" have less need to "act it out" in socially negative or health-endangering ways.
4. Focus and structure the discussion.	*"Let's get back to what you said about —."* *"Let's see if we can list the reasons."* *"In exactly what way has — been helpful to you?"*	Focusing brings the digressing patient back to the main discussion. You should listen for themes, even among the trivia. Similarities and differences in descriptions of events or persons by the patient should be pointed out. An overtalkative or aggressively hos-

Table continued on following page

T A B L E 1-2
Facilitative Verbal Responses *(Continued)*

Facilitative Response	Behavioral Examples	Theoretical Notes
	"Let's try to put things in order of priority." *"Go back to the beginning and tell me step by step."* *"Let's go over the choices you have."* *"I won't be giving you advice but if we carefully look at your options together, I think you will have a better sense of what you need to do next."* *"WHAT happened then?"* *"WHERE was that?"* *"WHEN did you become aware?"* *"HOW did that make you feel?"* Avoid "WHY?" questions because they tend to make people feel defensive.	tile patient may present a special challenge. It may be difficult to collect relevant data in a reasonable time period unless you firmly focus on one idea at a time. Remember that all behavior has meaning. Try to determine the reason for the overtalkativeness or hostility to reduce or diffuse it. Courteously interrupt with verbal and nonverbal cues when the discussion persistently wanders. Anxiety may make it difficult for a patient to focus on a particular topic for any length of time and your persistence with that topic may impede communication. Recognize that some patients use symbolic language or vague generalities to discuss anxiety-laden information.

		Try to help the patient organize what is being said. Often a patient has no idea where to begin to deal with the problems, especially if a number of unmet needs exist.
		Closed-ended questions, worded so that they can be answered with one or two words, are sometimes appropriate in structuring the discussion or filling gaps in the data.
		Help the patient delineate the collaborative role of the nurse and the active participation and basic responsibility of self in his/her own care.
5. Restate to clarify, validate or confront inconsistencies.	*"Am I clear that you said __?"* *"Could you go over that again?"* *"Let's see if I have that right. You said __."* *"In other words, you want to __."* *"Did you really mean __ when you said __?"*	Restatement conveys a strong message that what the patient says is important, and it conveys empathy. State the implied when the patient makes vague hints. Clarification helps both you and the patient understand what has been communicated in greater depth. Voicing doubts and using gentle confrontation to point out discrepancies promotes realistic thinking in greater depth.

Table continued on following page

T A B L E 1-2
Facilitative Verbal Responses (Continued)

Facilitative Response	Behavioral Examples	Theoretical Notes
	"What about __?"	
	"You said __ but now you are saying __?"	
	"Let's see. You did __ but you say __. I don't understand."	
	"You were smiling when you said you are so discouraged. How come?"	
	"Do you really believe that?"	
6. Provide feedback, interpretation, and summary.	*"I have the feeling that talking about __ makes you uncomfortable. Am I right?"* *"I notice that whenever I mention __ you change the subject. Is there a reason for this that you would like to talk about?"* *"Let's explore alternatives."*	Feedback should be descriptive and focus on concrete behaviors. It should not be judgmental. Alternatives should be explored, but giving advice should be avoided. The patient should be continually encouraged to give you feedback.

Summarizing synthesizes. It emphasizes major points, highlights progress, confirms consensual validation, and reinforces important information. It may be in written as well as verbal form. A plan for problem solving is mutually agreed upon and a sense of closure is provided.

"It sounds like you really want to —. Am I correct?"

"I would like to review what I think I heard you say. Please correct me if I'm wrong."

"Let me summarize what has been said and tell you how I see what is going on in your life."

"Here is some information about — and a list of resources."

"We agreed that you would first — and then contact —. Am I correct?"

"It looks like we've identified the major problems facing you and we talked about how you might begin to tackle them. Do you have any questions?"

"It seems to me that some progress has been made today. What do you think?"

Pediatric Considerations

Patient Profile Data

Birth child, adopted
Primary caretaker

Past Personal Health Data

Type of delivery
Apgar score
Gestational age
Birth weight
Neonatal complications/interventions
Feeding history (i.e., breast or bottle fed, type of formula,
   introduction of solids)
Past vitamin or fluoride regimens
Developmental milestones (Table 1–3)

Life-Style Data

Nanny, day care, "latch-key" child
Nuclear family, blended family, single parent, kinship care,
   foster care
Number of siblings, birth order
Sleeping arrangements (own room, sleeps with others)

Health Management Data

Home safety (e.g., cleaning fluids and corrosives placed in
   high cabinets, electric sockets plugged, water tempera-
   ture lowered)
Emergency medical care, poison control telephone num-
   bers available to caretaker; ipecac in the home
Use of car seat or seat belts
Tobacco use by caretakers or others in the home
Preventive dental care
Dietary practices
Sleep patterns
Bowel habits
Past hemoglobin, lead screening
Exercise, sports
Type of fun or leisure time activities

TABLE 1-3
Developmental Landmarks

Age	Developmental Landmark
Two weeks	Lifts head while prone. Regards other's face.
Two months	Grasps rattle. Coos/Reciprocal vocalization. Follows object 180 degrees. Smiles responsively.
Four Months	Holds head and neck up to make 90 angle. Rolls prone to supine. Hands midline. Laughs. Squeals. Follows object past midline.
Six Months	No head lag if baby is pulled to sitting position by hand. Rolls from back to abdomen or vice versa. Sits with a little support (one hand). Bears weight. Reaches for object on table, raking pattern. Turns towards sounds. Babbles vowels. Smiles spontaneously.
Nine Months	Sits alone. Crawls. Pulls self to standing position. Stands holding to solid object (not human). Has pincer grasp. Tries to get toy just out of reach. Transfers block from hand to hand. Resists toy being pulled away. Says "Da-da," "Ma-ma." Initial anxiety towards strangers. Plays "peek-a-boo."
Twelve Months	Stands alone 2-3 seconds if outside support removed. Cruises—walks around holding onto furniture. Bangs 2 blocks together if held one in each hand. Imitates vocalizing heard in preceding minute. Has 2-word vocabulary. Waves bye-bye.

Table continued on following page

TABLE 1–3
Developmental Landmarks (Continued)

Age	Developmental Landmark
Fifteen Months	Walks well. Stoops to recover toys on floor. Tries to feel self. Uses "Da-da" and "Ma-ma" specifically and correctly. Has 4 to 6-word vocabulary. Indicates wants by pulling, pointing, or appropriate verbalization (not crying). Plays "pat-a-cake."
Eighteen Months	Walks up stairs with one hand held. Puts one block on another without it falling off. Rolls or tosses ball back to examiner. Drinks from cup without spilling too much; uses spoon. Assists in removing clothing. Has 6 to 10-word vocabulary. Knows 1 body part. Mimics household chores like sweeping, dusting, etc.
Two Years	Goes up and down stairs holding rail. Kicks ball in front of self without support. Balances 4 blocks on top of one another. Dumps small object out of bottle after demonstration. Scribbles spontaneously—purposeful marking of more than one stroke. Combines 2 words. Has 50-word vocabulary. Points correctly to 5 parts of body. Does simple tasks in house.
Two-and-one-half Years	Throws overhand with demonstration. Combines 2 words meaningfully (subjects/predicates). Names correctly one picture in book, e.g., cat.
Three Years	Alternates feet ascending stairs. Jumps in place. Pedals tricycle. Dumps small articles from bottle without demonstration. Copies circle. Uses sentences intelligible to strangers.

TABLE 1–3
Developmental Landmarks *(Continued)*

Age	Developmental Landmark
	Puts on clothing.
	Washes and dries hands.
	Knows name, sex, and age.
Four Years	Alternates feet descending stairs.
	Balances on 1 foot for 5 seconds.
	Builds bridge of 3 blocks after demonstration.
	Copies circles and cross.
	Identifies longer of 2 lines.
	Cuts/Pastes.
	Dresses with supervision.
	Plays with other children so they interact.
	Understands what to do when tired, cold, hungry.
	Knows first and last names.
Five Years	Hops 2 or more times.
	Imitates forward heel-to-toe walk.
	Catches ball thrown three feet.
	Draws 3-part man.
	Dresses without supervision.
	Recognizes colors 3/4.
Six Years	Performs backward heel-toe walk.
	Copies a square.
	Draws a man with 6 parts.
	Ties shoelaces.
	Recognizes letters.
	Writes name.
	Defines 6 single words, e.g., ball, lake, house.
	Names materials of which things are made, e.g., spoon, door.

Adapted from Records. Used by the New City Pediatric Group P.C.

Psychosocial Data

Means of disciplining, behavior problems at home or in school

Fears, nervous habits, means of coping with stress

What grade in school, academic performance satisfactory

Trouble with the law

Values re: sexual matters (i.e., in harmony or conflict with parents)

Guidelines for Obtaining a Child's Health History

Provide adolescents with privacy and confidentiality

2

The Physical Examination

TECHNIQUES OF PHYSICAL EXAMINATION

The four basic techniques in physical examination are:
Inspection
Palpation
Percussion
Auscultation

Palpation follows inspection except when examining the abdomen, in which case it follows percussion and auscultation to avoid distortion of bowel sounds.

Inspection

Inspection is the visual examination of the patient.

Guidelines for Effective Inspection

Be systematic.
Fully expose the area to be inspected; cover other body parts to respect the patient's modesty.
Use a good light, preferably natural light, which will not distort colors. Use tangential lighting, which casts shadows, to increase visibility of variations in the body surface.
Consider racial and ethnic variations in skin color and texture.

Maintain a comfortable room temperature, as skin color is
  affected by both heat and cold.
Observe color, shape, size, symmetry, position, and movement.
Compare bilateral structures for similarities and differences. Take advantage of time spent with the patient
  when obtaining the health history to begin to inspect exposed body parts.

Palpation

Palpation is the use of the hand to touch for the purpose of
determining temperature, moisture, size, shape, position, texture, consistency, and movement. It is also used to check pulses;
to elicit tenderness, guarding, and rebound tenderness; and to
check for distention and edema.

Types of Palpation
LIGHT PALPATION

Use: To check muscle tone and assess for tender-
                  ness

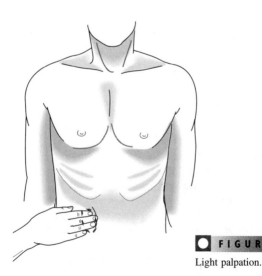

FIGURE 2-1

Light palpation.

Technique: Place the hand with fingers together parallel to the area being palpated. Press down 1 to 2 cm (½ to ¾ inch). Repeat in ever-widening circles until the area to be examined is covered (Fig. 2–1). Perform light palpation prior to deep palpation.

DEEP PALPATION

Use: To identify abdominal organs and abdominal masses

Technique: With the fingers together, approach the area to be examined at a 60 degree angle and use the pads and tips of the fingers of one hand to press in 4 cm (2 inches) (Fig. 2–2A). Be certain your fingernails are short to avoid injuring the patient's skin and keep in mind that deep palpation can be uncomfortable.

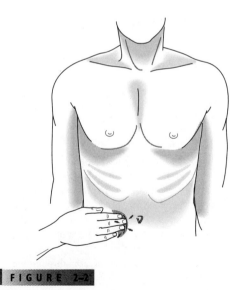

FIGURE 2–2

A, Single–handed deep palpation.

Illustration continued on following page

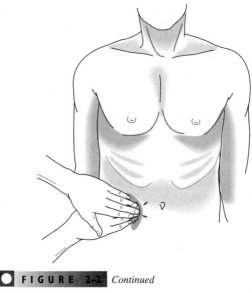

⬤ **F I G U R E   2–2**   *Continued*

B, Bimanual deep palpation.

For two-handed deep palpation proceed
as above but place the fingers of one hand on
top of those of the other (Fig. 2–2*B*).

Guidelines for Effective Palpation

Wash your hands before and after palpation.

Be aware that touching can cause embarrassment, and attempt to put the patient at ease: Explain all actions,
procedures, the "what, where, and why," as well as any
expected discomfort.

Make certain your hands are warm before placing them on
the patient's skin.

Ask the patient to take slow, deep breaths through the
mouth to decrease muscle tension, which can interfere
with palpation.

Palpate tender areas last; stop if pain occurs.

Use the pads of the fingers to assess texture, shape, size, and movement.

Use the back of the hand to check temperature.

Use the palmar or ulnar aspect of hand to assess vibrations.

Percussion

Percussion is the striking of the body surface with short, sharp strokes in order to produce palpable vibrations and characteristic sounds. It is used to determine the location, size, shape, and density of underlying structures; to detect the presence of air or fluid in a body space; and to elicit tenderness.

Types of Percussion

DIRECT PERCUSSION. Percussion in which one hand is used and the striking finger (plexor) of the examiner touches the surface being percussed.

Technique: Using sharp rapid movements from the wrist, strike the body surface to be percussed with the pads of two, three, or four fingers or with the pad of the middle finger alone. Primarily used to assess sinuses in the adult.

INDIRECT PERCUSSION. Percussion in which two hands are used and the plexor strikes the finger of the examiner's other hand, which is in contact with the body surface being percussed (pleximeter).

Technique: Place the distal portion of the hyperextended middle finger of the nondominant hand against the body surface to be percussed. Lift the other fingers and the rest of the hand so there is no contact of these parts with the patient's body surface.

Strike the pleximeter just behind the nail bed or at the distal interphalangeal joint with the tip of the middle finger of the dominant hand. Strike at a right angle to the pleximeter using a quick, sharp but relaxed wrist motion (Fig. 2–3). Withdraw the plexor immediately after the strike to avoid damping the vibration.

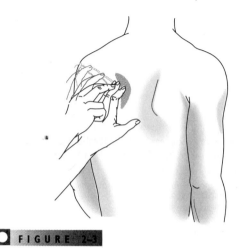

FIGURE 2-3

Indirect percussion.

Strike each area twice and then move to a new area. Use only the force necessary to produce a clear tone. Generally, the thicker the body wall in the area being percussed, the greater the force needed to produce a clear tone.

BLUNT PERCUSSION. Percussion in which the ulnar surface of the hand or fist is used in place of the fingers to strike the body surface, either directly or indirectly. In indirect blunt palpation the palm of the nondominant hand is placed flat against the body surface to be percussed and is struck by the ulnar surface of the fist of the dominant hand using a quick wrist motion (Fig. 2–4).

Percussion Sounds

Resonance:	A hollow sound like that produced by the normal lung
Hyperresonance:	A booming sound like that produced by an emphysematous lung
Tympany:	A musical or drum sound like that produced by the stomach and intestines

Dullness:	Thud sound produced by dense structures such as the liver, and enlarged spleen, or a full bladder
Flatness:	An extremely dull sound like that produced by very dense structures such as muscle or bone

As a general rule, the more air present in an area of percussion, the louder, deeper, and longer is the sound produced. Conversely, the more solid the area being percussed, the softer, higher, and shorter the sound produced.

Guidelines for Effective Percussion

Ensure a quiet environment.

Have the patient void before the examination.

Recognize that obesity can cause sounds to be muffled.

Make certain your hands are warm prior to touching the patient.

Maintain short fingernails.

Percuss from more resonant body areas to less resonant areas to facilitate detection of tone changes.

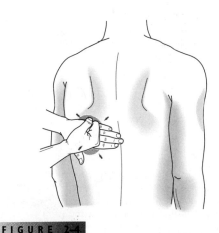

● FIGURE 2-4.

Indirect blunt percussion.

Use equal force on all areas to allow for accurate comparison.

Avoid percussing over ribs, scapulae, or other bony structures, otherwise only a dull sound will be heard.

Never use blunt percussion over the thorax of an elderly patient because of the risk of fracturing ribs.

Auscultation

Auscultation is listening to sounds produced inside the body. These include breath sounds, heart sounds, vascular sounds, and bowel sounds. Auscultation is used to detect the presence of normal and abnormal sounds and to assess them in terms of loudness, pitch, quality, frequency, and duration.

Guidelines for Effective Auscultation

Use an adequate stethoscope (Fig. 2–5):

- Tubing should be no longer than 12 to 14 inches (30 to 36 cm); longer tubing can distort sounds.
- Ear pieces should slope toward the nose and fit snugly but not to the point of pain.
- The bell of the stethoscope is used to auscultate low-pitched sounds such as extra heart sounds, murmurs and blood pressure. Hold the bell piece lightly against the skin surface when auscultating low-pitched sounds to avoid obliterating them.
- The diaphragm of the stethoscope is used to auscultate high-pitched sounds such as normal heart sounds, bowel sounds, and friction rubs. Place the full surface of the diaphragm flatly and firmly against the skin when auscultating high-pitched sounds.
- Avoid holding the diaphragm or bell with your thumb to avoid hearing your own pulse.

EQUIPMENT FOR PHYSICAL EXAMINATION

Basic equipment includes the following:

Tape measure and ruler marked in centimeters
Sphygmomanometer and cuff

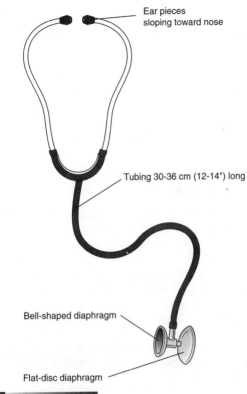

Ear pieces
sloping toward nose

Tubing 30-36 cm (12-14") long

Bell-shaped diaphragm

Flat-disc diaphragm

FIGURE 2-5

Stethoscope with bell and flat–disc diaphragm.

Stethoscope with a bell and diaphragm
Thermometer
Otoscope
Ophthalmoscope
Nasal speculum
Flashlight
Tongue blade
Reflex hammer

Tuning fork
Vision chart
Sharp object
Cotton balls
Vaginal speculum
Clean gloves
Lubricant
Materials for cytologic study and guaiac test reagents

Explain the use of each piece of equipment.

CONDUCTING THE PHYSICAL EXAMINATION

Introduce yourself, giving your name, title, and role, if not previously done during the history interview.

Ascertain if *cultural* norms exist relative to the conduct of the examination (e.g., male health care professionals may be prohibited from touching or examining females of traditional Arab, Hispanic, or other groups) and accommodate accordingly.

Recognize that a patient may feel anxious and embarrassed about being examined.

Act in a calm, confident, organized manner.

Avoid manifesting negative reactions, such as alarm or disgust.

Be sensitive to the patient's feelings.

Maintain a quiet environment free of interruptions and distractions.

Work in good lighting, natural if possible.

Ensure maximum privacy by draping the patient, closing doors, and pulling curtains.

Position the patient appropriately for the part of the body examined (Table 2–1).

Promote the patient's physical comfort: use warm hands and instruments and maintain a warm environment.

Keep the patient informed of what you are going to do and why.

Be systematic and follow a planned order of examination.

Work from the patient's right side, moving to the back and left as needed.

Be gentle and warn the patient of any expected discomfort.

Wear gloves for contact with any body fluid or open lesions.

Pay special attention to areas of the body about which the patient has current complaints or a history of problems.

Allow time for patient questions.

Document findings:

- Be accurate.
- Be concise
- Be organized.
- Use only accepted abbreviations.
- Avoid subjective terms such as normal, abnormal, good, or poor.
- Include both positive and negative findings.

Geriatric Considerations

Be alert to impaired vision and/or hearing and adjust communication techniques accordingly.

Perform the examination at a pace comfortable for the patient, providing rest periods as needed.

Require as few position changes as possible during the examination to prevent fatigue.

Direct the patient to change position slowly to protect against orthostatic hypotension and/or dizziness.

Be sure the room is warm and the patient is adequately covered because older patients tend to chill easily.

Use a low, wide examination table to promote mobility and prevent accidents.

Never leave a confused patient on the examining table unattended.

Use a step stool to aid the patient in getting safely on and off the examining table.

TABLE 2-1
Patient Positions for Physical Examination

Position	Illustration	Use	Notes
Sitting: back unsupported, legs dangling freely	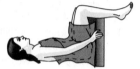	Measurement of vital signs. Examination of head, neck, chest, breasts, back, lungs, axillae, arms, and hands.	Use supine position with head elevated if patient is unable to tolerate sitting unsupported

Supine: lying on back with legs extended

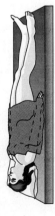

Examination of head, neck, chest, breasts, lungs, axillae, arms, hands, abdomen, legs, and feet

Use a pillow under the head and the knees if needed to make the patient comfortable and to relax abdominal muscles; elevate the patient's head if dyspnea occurs

Dorsal recumbent: lying on back with knees flexed, hips externally rotated and small pillow under the head

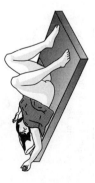

Examination of head, neck, chest, breasts, lungs, heart, and axillae

Patients with certain cardiac, pulmonary, or joint problems may be unable to assume or maintain this position

Table continued on following page

T A B L E   2–1
Patient Positions for Physical Examination (Continued)

Position	Illustration	Use	Notes
Lithotomy: lying on back, buttocks at edge of table, feet in stirrups		Examination of female genitalia and rectum	As for dorsal recumbent
Sims: lying on side with upper leg flexed in front of body and lower arm beind the body		Examination of rectum and vagina	Patients with joint limitations may be unable to assume the Sims position

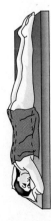

Prone: lying on abdomen, face to side

Examination of hip extension

As for dorsal recumbent

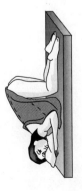

Knee–chest: kneeling with head and arms down to create a 90 degree angle between torso and hips

Examination of the rectum

As for dorsal recumbent; special tables are available that support the patient in knee–chest position

Pediatric Considerations

Allow the child to stand or sit on the caretaker's lap for as much of the examination as possible before moving the child to the examining table.

Position the caretaker within the child's view; allow comfort measures that do not interfere with the examination.

Approach the patient gently; give firm directions; do not allow choices where there are none (e.g., "Do you want to open your mouth?" as compared to "Please open your mouth now.").

Explain directions/actions in developmentally appropriate language; distract infants.

Allow the child to handle equipment (stethoscope, otoscope) to reduce fear and foster feelings of control.

Save those aspects of examination likely to induce crying for last.

Restrain firmly as needed, the general rule being: restrain the joint above and the joint below the part to be immobilized. Restrain the head by extending the child's arms above the head and firmly pressing them toward the midline.

Provide adolescents with privacy and confidentiality; consider allowing a "buddy" to be present where appropriate.

3
The General Physical Assessment Survey

The general survey is a preliminary assessment of the individual that provides the nurse with an initial, overall impression of the whole patient. It provides essential information about the patient's behavior, outstanding physical characteristics, and general health status.

Information gathered about the patient's health includes subjective data (symptoms) elicited from questions asked (by the nurse), and objective data (signs) identified by observations and measurements.

The general survey is initiated as soon as the patient is encountered, continues through the health history interview, and is followed by the complete physical assessment. Documentation consists of a short summary statement, usually in the form of a paragraph.

EXAMPLE: T.L. is a short, obese Asian American male who appears to be his reported age of 52 years. His skin color is normal and there are no signs of acute distress. He is well developed and well groomed, and his dress is neat and appropriate. He is alert and oriented, speaks clearly and slowly, and is cooperative. He sits erect, is attentive, and maintains eye contact.

Height: 5 feet, 4 inches (162.56 cm); weight: 194 lbs
  (88.19 kg)
T: 98°F; P: 84; R: 16; BP: 134/86

The general survey focuses on the assessment of the
following major areas:

Overall physical appearance
Behavior
Body development and movement
Height and weight
Vital signs

Equipment required includes the following:

Floor model platform balance scale with height measuring
  attachment
Tape measure
Thermometer
Stethoscope
Sphygmomanometer and cuff
Watch with a second hand
Lubricant

OVERALL PHYSICAL APPEARANCE

Age

Questions

What is your current age?

Procedure/Technique/Findings

Compare apparent age to reported or documented age.
  Note physiologic signs of aging such as changes in skin,
  gait, posture, muscle strength, and mental alertness.

Normal Findings	**Abnormal Findings**
Overall appearance of the patient is consistent with chronological age	Patient appears younger or older than chronological age

Level of Consciousness

Also, see Chapter 5, Mental Status Assessment.

Questions

Routine questions posed during the health history interview often reveal the desired information. When necessary ask the following:

- What is your first and last name?
- What is today's date?
- What is the name of this place?

Procedure/Technique/Findings

Note whether the patient is alert and oriented to time,
place, and person.
Note the level of understanding of questions.
Check the ability to follow directions by asking the patient
to squeeze your fingers.
Note the ability to answer questions and to follow
instructions.

Normal Findings	Abnormal Findings
Patient is awake, alert and aware of the environment	Patient is lethargic and unaware of the environment
Oriented to time, place and person	Disoriented to time, place, and/or person
Pays attention to questions, responds quickly, and answers appropriately	Unable to answer questions appropriately
Follows instructions	Unable to follow instructions

Signs Of Distress

Questions

Ask the patient to validate and/or clarify nursing observations related to noted signs of distress.
When necessary ask the following:

- When did the signs or symptoms begin?

- What factors precipitated or aggravated the signs or symptoms?
- Does anything bring relief?

Procedure/Technique/Findings

Note any signs or symptoms of physical and/or emotional distress, such as pain or difficulty breathing.

Determine whether distress is related to a condition that requires further assessment and immediate intervention.

Normal Findings

Absence of signs and symptoms of distress

Abnormal Findings

Presence of dyspnea, wheezing, stridor, restlessness, cyanosis, facial grimacing, guarding of a body part, writhing, crying, moaning, fidgeting, diaphoresis, cold moist palms, bleeding

Sexual Development

Questions

None.

Procedure/Technique/Findings

Note the presence of facial hair, breast size, and characteristics of the voice with regard to age and gender.

Consider sociocultural variations (e.g., facial hirsutism is common in Caucasian women, occurring in 40% of this population, and is uncommon in Japanese women).

Normal Findings

Appropriate for age and gender

Abnormal Findings

Early or retarded sexual development

Presence of excessive breast development in the male (gynecomastia), abnormal facial hair in the female

Skin Color and Condition

Also, see Chapter 6, Assessment of the Skin, Hair, and Nails.

Questions

None.

Procedure/Technique/Findings

Note the general color, temperature, and presence of edema and/or lesions on exposed body parts (e.g., face, hands, and arms).

Use good lighting.

Consider sociocultural variations (e.g., keloids are more common in African Americans).

Normal Findings	Abnormal Findings
Pink tones in light-skinned persons, and light to brown or olive tones in dark-skinned persons	Presence of flushing, pallor, cyanosis, or yellowing
	Areas of increased pigmentation, erythema, or echymosis
Warm or cool temperature	Hot or cold temperature
Absence of edema	Presence of edema
Absence of lesions	Presence of lesions (see Table 6–1)

Facial Features

Questions

None.

Procedure/Technique/Findings

Note size and symmetry of features.
Note facial mobility.
Note presence of edema and/or abnormal facial movement.

Normal Findings	Abnormal Findings
Symmetry of features	Asymmetry of features
Absence of enlarged features	Distorted features

Bilateral movement	Unilateral movement
	Inability to close eye
Absence of edema	Periorbital edema
Absence of drooping/ptosis	Drooping/ptosis
	Decreased blink rate
	Staring, expressionless, mask-like face
Absence of abnormal movements	Tics, oral-facial dyskinesia

Personal Hygiene and Dress

Questions

Ask the patient questions to clarify observations made regarding dress and personal hygiene. Long sleeves or a wide-brimmed hat may be worn to protect against the sun. Oversized clothing may indicate a recent weight loss. Excessive clothing may indicate an intolerance to cold. Untied shoes may indicate pedal edema or pain, or difficulty completing fine motor tasks. A belt with new holes may indicate ascites or weight gain. Incorrectly buttoned clothing may indicate a visual deficit. An unkempt appearance may indicate depression or physical illness.

Procedure/Technique/Findings

Note whether clothing is appropriate to weather, occasion, age group, culture, life-style, and socioeconomic group.
Note whether skin, hair, and nails are neat and clean, and whether makeup is appropriate.
Note the patient's level of concern for appearance.
Note signs of neglect with regard to personal hygiene.
Note indications of inability to perform self-care.
Note whether equal attention is paid to hygiene and grooming on both sides of the body.

Normal Findings	*Abnormal Findings*
Dress is clean, neat, fits properly, and is appropriate	Clothing is unclean, inappropriate, and/or fits poorly

Skin, hair, and nails are clean and neat	Skin, hair, and/or nails are unkempt
Makeup is appropriate	Face is unshaven in previously clean-shaven male
	Absence of makeup in a previously made up female, inappropriate makeup

Body and Breath Odors

Questions

None.

Procedure/Technique/Findings

Note the presence of general body and/or breath odors. Consider sociocultural variations (e.g., Asians and Native Americans normally have at most mild body odor; African Americans and Caucasians have a strong body odor; ethnic food preferences may affect breath odors).

Normal Findings	Abnormal Findings
Absence of body and breath odors in persons with typical American sociocultural hygienic values (absence of other than normal body odor in persons with sociocultural hygienic values other than typical American)	Presence of halitosis or foul odor
	Smell of alcohol on the breath
	Acetone, sweet, or ammonia odor to breath
	Body odor, odor of urine or feces
	Excessive use of colognes or perfumes

Obvious Deformities

Questions

Is the deformity congenital or acquired?

Procedure/Technique/Findings

Note any apparent physical deformity.

Normal Findings	*Abnormal Findings*
Absence of physical deformity	Amputated or missing extremities, digits, and/or features
	Underdeveloped extremities

BEHAVIOR

Mood, Manner and Affect

Questions

None.

Procedure/Technique/Findings

Note the patient's anxiety level.
Note the patient's mood, affect, and emotional tone.
Note and compare the patient's behavior and verbal responses.

Normal Findings	*Abnormal Findings*
Mild anxiety, comfortable in situation	Moderate to extreme anxiety, nervousness, restlessness, agitation, crying
Cooperative attitude	Uncooperative, angry, aggressive, or combative attitude
Attentive	Inattentive
Affect and mood appropriate to the situation	Affect and/or mood inappropriate to situation
	Apathetic, depressed, euphoric, stooped posture
	Bizarre mannerisms (e.g., repeated patting or rubbing of body parts)

Facial Expressions

Questions

None.

Procedure/Technique/Findings

Note the patient's facial expressions while conversing and at rest.

Note eye contact with you and with others.

Consider sociocultural values.

Normal Findings	**Abnormal Findings**
Facial expression is appropriate to discussion and situation	Flat, dejected, blank, exaggerated, or inappropriate facial expression
	Facial trembling, staring, or excessive blinking
Maintains eye contact as appropriate for cultural background [i.e., some cultures (Asian, Arab, Native American) consider direct eye contact as impolite or aggressive]	Absence of eye contact

Speech and Speech Patterns

Questions

None.

Procedure/Technique/Findings

Note speech pattern, pace, vocabulary, sentence structure, and thought pattern.

Note quality, tone, clarity, and strength of voice.

Note speech defects.

Consider sociocultural variations (e.g., appropriate use of words and/or foreign accent in patients for whom English is a second language).

Normal Findings	**Abnormal Findings**
Even, moderately paced speech	Slow, fast, halting, deliberate, interrupted, slurred, or garbled speech
Clear, understandable voice	Soft, loud, weak, hoarse, monotone, high-pitched voice

Appropriate use of words	Ideas conveyed in a disorganized manner
	Aphasia, dysphasia
	Inappropriate vocabulary
Absence of speech defects	Stuttering, lisping

BODY DEVELOPMENT AND MOVEMENT

Stature

Questions

What is your current height?
How tall are your parents and siblings?

Procedure/Technique/Findings

Note the patient's general height.
Consider sociocultural variations (e.g., Caucasian American men average approximately 0.5 inches (1.27 cm) greater height than African American men; Native Americans, Mexican Americans, and Asian Americans tend to be shorter than both Caucasian and African Americans).
Height tends to be directly proportionate to socioeconomic status for all ethnic groups.

| *Normal Findings* | *Abnormal Findings* |
| Height correlates with average for age, sex, and/or genetic predisposition | Taller or shorter than average for age, sex, and/or genetic expectation |

Body Build and Type

Questions

None.

Procedure/Technique/Findings

Note general body build and type.

Note fat distribution pattern.
Consider sociocultural variations (e.g., amount of body fat tends to be inversely proportionate to socioeconomic status).

Normal Findings	*Abnormal Findings*
Size and general shape are average, slender, lanky, trim, muscular, or stocky	Poorly developed musculature and inadequate fat
	Flabbiness
	Emaciation, obesity
	Uneven distribution of fat, truncal obesity, "moon facies"

Symmetry and Proportion

Questions

What is your current height?

Procedure/Technique/Findings

Note general arrangement and symmetry of body parts.
Note general proportions of body and length of limbs.
Ask the patient to spread arms to determine length of span.
Compare arm span with the patient's height.
Consider decreasing height in the elderly.
Consider sociocultural variations (e.g., African Americans have longer extremities than Caucasian Americans).

Normal Findings	*Abnormal Findings*
Size and shape of body parts are symmetrical	Asymmetry of size and shape of body parts
Arm span is proportionate with height	Long limbs in relation to height

Posture and Position

Questions

None.

Procedure/Technique/Findings

Note the patient's posture while standing and sitting.
Note positions assumed.
Consider the patient's age.

Normal Findings	Abnormal Findings
Stands and sits straight with good body alignment	Posture bent, stooped, stiff, tense, rigid, or overly relaxed
Posture relaxed	Slumped shoulders, rigid spine and neck, sway back
	Forward leaning position with arms extended, inability to lie down, lies still without moving, lies with knees drawn up, writhes in bed, unable to bend knees and neck without pain, hunched position, dystonia.

Gait

Questions

None.

Procedure/Technique/Findings

Ask the patient to walk a short distance toward and away from you (if the patient was not observed entering the room).
Note speed, smoothness, and style of gait.
Note use of assistive devices and prosthetic limbs.

Normal Findings	Abnormal Findings
Smooth, coordinated, even, steady, secure gait	Stiff, staggering, stumbling, unsteady, uncoordinated gait
	Limping, dragging, extension, circumduction of leg
	Fast, shuffling, accelerating gait with difficulty stopping

Looks down at ground while walking

Use of cane, walker, brace, crutches, prosthetic limb

Good balance | Loss of balance

Arms swing freely | Increased, decreased, asymmetrical arm swing

Motor Activity

Questions

None.

Procedure/Technique/Findings

Note voluntary and involuntary movements of limbs and face.

Note symmetry of movement.

Normal Findings	Abnormal Findings
Coordinated, smooth, symmetrical voluntary movement	Asymmetrical movement
	Immobility, paralysis, paresis of body parts
Absence of involuntary movement	Slow, writhing, continuous movement
	Sudden, rapid, jerky, bizarre, repeated movement
	Involuntary, purposeless movement
	Tremors at rest, tremors with voluntary movement
	Fasciculations, tics, seizures, athetosis, chorea

WEIGHT AND HEIGHT

Weight

Questions

What is your usual weight?

Procedure/Technique/Findings

Use a standard balance beam platform scale (Fig. 3–1A).

Determine that the scale is balanced by checking to see that the balance bar remains centered when the weights are placed on the zero mark. Adjust as necessary.

Floor models are used for patients who are able to stand unassisted.

Bed scales or chair scales are used for patients who are immobilized or unable to stand (Fig. 3–1B). (Specialty beds are available that allow the patient to be weighed in bed.)

Consider sociocultural variations (e.g., bone density in both women and men is greater in African Americans than in Caucasian Americans; African American women tend to weigh more than Caucasian American women; and Asian Americans tend to weigh less than Caucasian Americans).

FLOOR MODEL

Explain the procedure to the patient.

Assess the patient's ability to stand without assistance.

Instruct the patient to remove shoes and any excessive or heavy outerwear.

Place a clean paper towel on the platform and assist the patient onto the scale.

Instruct the patient to stand in the center of the platform, to avoid leaning on the scale, and to remain still.

Slide the weights down the balance bar until the tip of the balance bar remains centered.

Read the patient's weight by adding the numbers indicated by the position of the weights.

Record the patient's weight in pounds (lbs) or kilograms (kg). (Pounds may be converted to kilograms by dividing by 2.2.)

Compare the patient's actual weight with the recommended range for the patient's sex, height, and frame size (see Appendix 1).

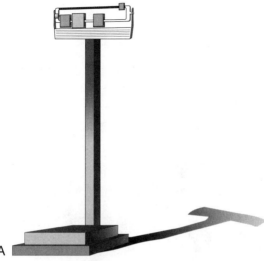

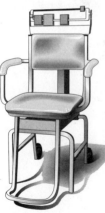

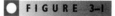

● FIGURE 3–1

A, Standard balance beam platform scale. *B*, Chair scale.

A

B

Normal Findings	*Abnormal Findings*
Weight within desired range for sex, height, and frame size (see Appendix 1)	Weight above or below desired range for sex, height, and frame size (see Appendix 1)

Height

Questions

How tall are your parents and siblings?

Procedure/Technique/Findings

Use the sliding, vertical measuring bar attached to the floor model scale when the patient is able to stand without assistance (Fig. 3–2).

A tape measure or measuring stick attached to the wall may also be utilized.

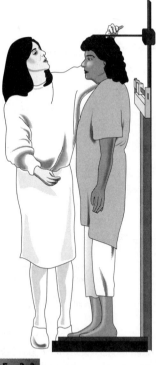

◯ FIGURE 3–2

Use of the sliding, vertical measuring bar attached to a floor model scale to measure patient's height.

The height of an immobilized patient may be measured by marking the top of the head and the heels on the sheet while the patient is stretched out in a supine position. The distance between the marks is measured with a measuring tape.

Arm span rather than height may be measured in patients with marked osteoporosis and spinal curvature as well as in patients confined to bed or a wheelchair. Measure arm span by directing the patient to hold his or her arms straight out to the sides of the body and measure from tip of middle finger of one hand to tip of middle finger of the other hand.

VERTICAL MEASURING BAR OR WALL MEASUREMENT

Explain the procedure to the patient.

Assess the patient's ability to stand unassisted.

Instruct the patient to remove his or her shoes, face away from the balance beam, place the feet together centered on the platform, stand straight, look straight ahead, and allow the arms to hang freely at sides.

Instruct the patient being measured against a wall to place heels, buttocks, shoulders, and head against the wall.

Slide the measuring bar up so that the top is above the patient's head.

Extend the horizontal rod and lower the measuring bar until the rod rests lightly on top of the patient's head at a right angle to the measuring bar.

Read the patient's height by noting the number displayed where the top part of the measuring bar slides down into the bottom stationary part.

Read the height of a patient measured against a wall by noting where a ruler or straight object, resting on top of the patient's head, touches the wall at a right angle.

Record the height in inches (") or centimeters (cm). (Inches may be converted into centimeters by multiplying by 2.54.)

Consider age-related factors (e.g., decreased height related to postural changes and shortening of the spine).

Normal Findings	*Abnormal Findings*
Height within average range for sex, age, and genetic expectation	Taller or shorter than average range for sex, age, and genetic expectation

Geriatric Considerations

Additional History Questions

Is there a difference between your current diet and your diet at midlife?

What factors affect diet (e.g., tooth loss, dental problems, decreased smell, taste or saliva, stomach or bowel problems, chronic disease, depression, reduced social contact, difficulty shopping or cooking, financial restraints, multiple medications or drugs)?

Clinical Notes

Decreasing physical activity may necessitate a lower daily caloric intake.

Common medications can interact with certain foods, affect appetite, or change the body's nutritional requirements. Assess medications carefully.

Unintentional weight loss of 5% or more in 1 month, 7.5% or more in 3 months, or 10% more in 6 months in the older patient may be an ominous sign of serious underlying disease and must be investigated.

VITAL SIGNS

Temperature

Questions

Have you had an elevated temperature recently? Onset? Duration? Frequency? Associated with a known illness?

Procedure/Technique/Findings

Consider time of day, age, and activity prior to measurement.

Determine the best method of measurement for the patient and select the appropriate thermometer (Fig. 3–3).

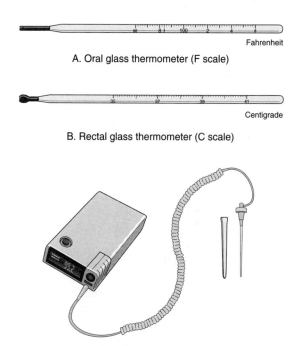

Fahrenheit

A. Oral glass thermometer (F scale)

Centigrade

B. Rectal glass thermometer (C scale)

C. Electronic thermometer

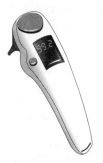

D. Tympanic thermometer

FIGURE 3-3

Types of thermometers. *A,* Oral glass thermometer. *B,* Rectal glass thermometer. *C,* Electronic thermometer. *D,* Tympanic thermometer.

Avoid oral measurement of temperature in patients who
  are disoriented, confused, comatose, or unable to keep
  the mouth closed, and in those who are intubated, have
  chills, have a history of convulsions, or have had recent
  oral surgery and/or are receiving oxygen via a face mask.
Delay oral measurement of temperature for at least 15
  minutes following gum chewing, ingestion of hot or cold
  fluids, and/or smoking.
Avoid rectal measurement of temperature in patients with
  recent rectal surgery, hemorrhoids, and/or position limitations.
Utilize axillary measurement of temperature when oral,
  rectal, and tympanic measurements are contraindicated.

ORAL ELECTRONIC THERMOMETER

Explain the procedure to the patient.
Place the patient in a comfortable position.
Charge and place a disposable cover on the oral probe.
Place sublingually and leave in place until the signal indi-
  cates completion (approximately 30 seconds).
Read the digital display.
Record the reading.

ORAL GLASS THERMOMETER

Explain the procedure to the patient.
Place the patient in a comfortable position.
Cleanse and shake down the glass mercury thermometer to
  95°F (35°C) or below.
Ask the patient to open the mouth and raise the tongue.
Place the tip of the thermometer under the tongue in one
  of the sublingual pockets at the base of the tongue.
Instruct the patient to keep the mouth and lips closed, to
  hold the thermometer with the lips, and to avoid biting
  down.
Leave the thermometer in place for 3 to 5 minutes.
Remove the thermometer and read the mercury at eye
  level.
Record the reading.

RECTAL ELECTRONIC THERMOMETER

Explain the procedure to the patient.

Maintain the patient's privacy.

Place a disposable cover on the rectal probe. Insert rectally, and wait for the completion signal.

Read the digital display.

Record the reading.

RECTAL GLASS THERMOMETER

Explain the procedure to the patient.

Maintain the patient's privacy.

Cleanse and shake down the mercury glass thermometer to 95°F (35°C) or below.

Lubricate the bulb with a water-soluble lubricant.

Place the patient in a side-lying position with the upper leg flexed.

Apply disposable gloves.

Insert the tip of the thermometer gently for a distance of approximately 1 to 1.5 inches (2.54 to 3.81 cm).

Hold the thermometer in place for 3 minutes.

Remove the thermometer, wipe off with a tissue, and read the mercury at eye level.

Record the reading.

AXILLARY TEMPERATURE MONITORING

Explain the procedure to the patient.

Maintain the patient's privacy.

Cleanse and shake down the mercury glass thermometer to 95°F (35°C) or below.

Expose the patient's arm and shoulder.

Place the patient in a supine or sitting position.

Raise the patient's arm and place the tip of the thermometer in the center of the axilla.

Lower the arm and position it across the chest.

Leave the thermometer in place for 5 to 10 minutes.

Remove the thermometer and read the mercury at eye level.

Record the reading.

TYMPANIC TEMPERATURE MONITORING

Explain the procedure to the patient.

Place the patient in a supine or sitting position.

Gently place the covered tip of the probe into the auditory canal.

Activate the starter and read the digital display in approximately 2 seconds.

Normal Findings	*Abnormal Findings*
Oral temperature 97° to 100° F (36° to 37.8° C)	Fever (hyperthermia, pyrexia): >100° F (37.8° C) orally
	Hypothermia: <97° F (36° C) orally
Rectal temperature 98° to 101° F (37° to 38.8° C)	Fever: >101° F (38.8° C) rectally
	Hypothermia: <98° F (37° C) rectally.
Axillary temperature 96° to 99° F (35° to 36.8° C)	Fever: >99° F (36.8° C) axillary
	Hypothermia: <96° F (35° C)
Tympanic temperature	Fever: / Hypothermia: { Refer to oral or rectal norms depending on which is selected on the tympanic thermometer
	Chills, shivering, diaphoresis

Pulse

Questions

Are you currently taking any medications that affect your heart?

Procedure/Technique/Findings

Consider the patient's age, presence of fever or pain, factors that stimulate the sympathetic nervous system (fear, anger, stress), and factors that stimulate the parasympathetic nervous system (vomiting, suctioning, medications, caffeine ingestion and physical training).

Consider and select the appropriate site and method of measurement (Fig. 3–4).

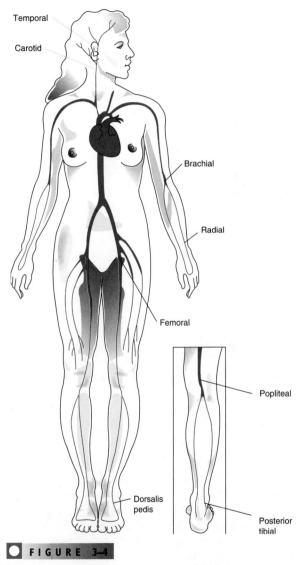

Temporal

Carotid

Brachial

Radial

Femoral

Popliteal

Dorsalis pedis

Posterior tibial

FIGURE 3-4

Major sites for palpating the pulse.

RADIAL PULSE

Explain the procedure to the patient.

Position the patient comfortably with the forearm supported, the palm facing down, and the wrist slightly extended.

Locate the radial artery on the thumb side of the inner surface of the wrist.

Use the pads of the middle three fingers to compress the radial artery against the bone and then slowly release it until the pulse is felt.

Count the pulse rate for one full minute using a watch with a second hand.

Note the rhythm of the pulse.

Note the quality (e.g., full, weak, bounding, thready) of the pulse.

Note the equality of the radial pulses on both sides.

Record the pulse rate, rhythm, quality, and equality.

Avoid using the thumb to palpate the pulse.

Delay measurement of the pulse for 10 minutes following activity.

ALTERNATE TECHNIQUE—RADIAL PULSE UTILIZING A DOPPLER ULTRASOUND

Utilize a Doppler ultrasound stethoscope to auscultate the pulse if the radial pulse is not manually palpable (Fig. 3–5).

Explain the procedure to the patient.

Connect the stethoscope (headset) to the ultrasound probe (transducer).

Position the patient comfortably with the forearm supported and the palm facing upward.

Locate the radial artery on the thumb side of the inner surface of the wrist.

Apply a thin layer of conductive gel to the skin over the radial artery or directly to the probe (transducer).

Gently place the probe (transducer) over the radial artery touching the skin at a 45 to 90 degree angle.

Turn the On–Off switch on the Doppler to the On position
  and adjust the volume control.

Listen for a pulsating or wavelike swooshing sound.

Move the probe slightly while maintaining skin contact
  until the sound is detected.

Count the pulse rate for one full minute using a watch
  with a second hand.

Clean the gel from the skin and instrument.

Record the fact that a Doppler was used, the pulse rate,
  and the character and intensity of the sound.

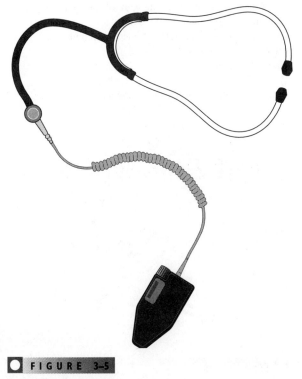

⬤ FIGURE 3-5

Doppler ultrasound stethoscope.

APICAL PULSE

Auscultate the apical pulse routinely or when the patient is known to have an arrhythmia and/or is on cardiac medication.

Delay measurement of the apical pulse for 10 minutes following activity.

Explain the procedure to the patient.

Maintain the patient's privacy.

Place the patient in a comfortable position with access to the chest.

Locate the apex of the heart at the fifth intercostal space in line with the left mid-clavicle.

Place the stethoscope over the apex of the heart and auscultate the apical pulse (Fig. 3–6).

Count the apical pulse rate for one full minute using a watch with a second hand.

Note the rhythm of the apical pulse.

Record the apical pulse rate and rhythm.

Clean the stethoscope between patients.

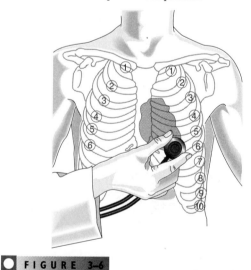

● F I G U R E 3–6

Position of the stethoscope to obtain an apical pulse.

Normal Findings	**Abnormal Findings**
Radial pulse rate: 50 to 90 beats/minute	Tachycardia: radial pulse rate >90 beats/minute
	Bradycardia: radial pulse rate <50 beats/minute
Regular rhythm	Irregular radial pulse
Quality is full, easily palpated, and equal bilaterally	Weak, thready, feeble, bounding, asymmetrical radial pulses
Apical pulse rate: 50 to 90 beats/minute	Tachycardia, bradycardia
Regular rhythm	Irregular rhythm

Respirations

Questions

Have you had any respiratory tract infections?
Do you have any allergies that affect your breathing?
Do you have a history of respiratory disorders (e.g., asthma)?

Procedure/Technique/Findings

Consider the patient's age, presence of fever or pain, current illness, and medications.

Observe respirations following measurement of the radial pulse.

Avoid making the patient aware that respirations are being evaluated by keeping your fingers on the radial artery.

Observe a complete respiratory cycle prior to counting by noting the rise and fall of the chest, or by feeling the rise and fall with your hand on the patient's chest or upper abdomen.

Use a watch with a second hand.

Count the number of complete respiratory cycles in 30 seconds and multiply by 2 if respirations are unlabored and regular.

Count the number of complete respiratory cycles in 1 minute if respirations are labored and irregular.

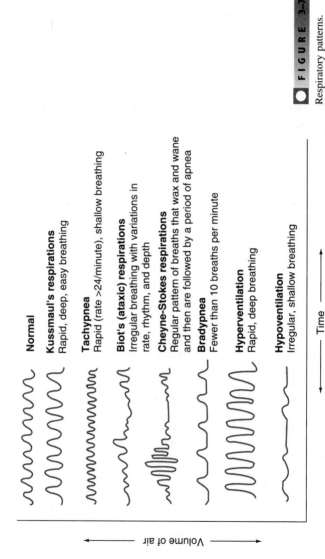

FIGURE 3–7
Respiratory patterns.

Note the depth of the respirations.
Note the rhythm and pattern of the respirations (Fig. 3–7).
Note the effort required for respiration and the use of
  accessory muscles.
Record the respiratory rate, depth, and rhythm.

Normal Findings	*Abnormal Findings*
Respiratory rate 12 to 20/minute	Tachypnea: respiratory rate >20/minute
	Bradypnea: respiratory rate <12/minute
Relaxed, effortless, regular respiration	Labored (dyspnea), irregular rhythm
	Restlessness, anxiety, wheezing, stridor
	Shallow (hypopnea), deep (hyperpnea) respirations
	Hyperventilation, hypoventilation, Cheyne–Stokes or Kussmaul respirations
Symmetrical chest wall expansion	Asymmetrical chest expansion
	Use of accessory muscles of respiration, puffed cheeks, pursed lips, muscle retraction, nasal flaring

See chapter 14, Assessment of the Chest and Lungs, for
alterations in breath sounds.

See chapter 6, Assessment of the Skin, Hair, and Nails, for
alterations in skin and nail color.

Blood Pressure

Questions

Do you have any history of high or low blood pressure?
Are you currently taking any antihypertensive medications
  or diuretics (blood pressure pills or water pills)?
Do you have any history of fainting?

Procedure/Technique/Findings

Consider the patient's age, sex, race, weight, emotional status, presence of pain, time of day, and medications.

Consider sociocultural variations (e.g., African Americans have a greater incidence, severity, and earlier age of onset of hypertension than Caucasian Americans).

Delay blood pressure measurement by at least 30 minutes after the patient has exercised, smoked, or ingested caffeine.

Refrain from using the arm on the side of a mastectomy, intravenous infusion, or hemodialysis access site.

Allow the patient to rest 5 minutes prior to initiating procedure.

Explain the procedure to the patient.

Position the patient in a comfortable sitting or lying position with the forearm supported at the level of the heart and the palm facing upward.

Expose the upper arm by removing any clothing and/or by rolling loose clothing completely out of the way. (Avoid any constriction of the arm with clothing that is rolled up.)

Select a cuff (Fig. 3–8) that is intact and is the appropriate size for the patient. (The cuff should cover two-thirds of the upper arm and completely encircle the arm.)

Locate the brachial artery on the inner aspect of the elbow by palpation.

Wrap the deflated cuff securely, evenly, and snugly around the arm, with the center of the cuff positioned directly over the brachial artery and the lower edge of the cuff positioned approximately 1 inch (2.54 cm) above the antecubital fossa.

Position the table model, mercury manometer at eye level.

Estimate the systolic pressure by palpating the brachial artery while inflating the cuff and noting the reading on the manometer at which the pulse disappears (estimated systolic pressure).

Deflate the cuff and wait 30 seconds.

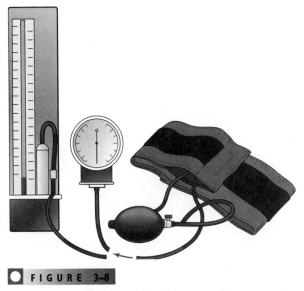

FIGURE 3–8

Blood pressure cuff with aneroid and mercury sphygnomanometers.

Place the stethoscope over the brachial artery with light, firm pressure (Fig. 3–9). Avoid any contact with clothing or the cuff.

Inflate the cuff to 30 mmHg above the estimated systolic pressure.

Deflate the cuff slowly and steadily at an approximate rate of 2 to 3 mmHg per second.

Note the readings on the manometer at which the first consecutive sounds are heard (Korotkoff I) and at which the sound disappears (Korotkoff V).

Continue to deflate and remove the cuff.

Record these readings as the systolic and diastolic pressures, respectively.

Repeat this procedure on the same arm if blood pressure is elevated. Wait at least 30 seconds between measurements.

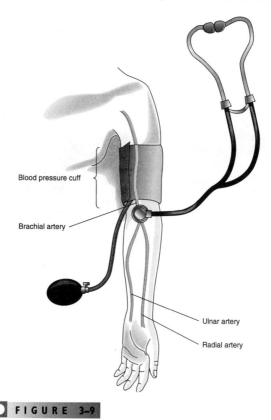

Blood pressure cuff

Brachial artery

Ulnar artery

Radial artery

○ FIGURE 3-9

Blood pressure cuff in place with stethoscope positioned over the brachial artery.

Note differences.

Repeat this procedure on the other arm.

Note differences.

Repeat this procedure in the sitting, lying, and standing positions if the patient has a history of hypertension or syncope or is on antihypertensive medication.

Note differences.

Clean the stethoscope between patients.

ALTERNATE TECHNIQUE—BLOOD PRESSURE MEASUREMENT UTILIZING DOPPLER ULTRASOUND

Utilize a Doppler ultrasound stethoscope to amplify sound and auscultate the blood pressure when a standard stethoscope is ineffective (e.g., in obese patients and those in shock).

Explain the procedure to the patient.

Proceed as above.

Locate the brachial artery on the inner aspect of the elbow by palpation.

Wrap the deflated cuff around the arm as above.

Apply a thin layer of conductive gel to the skin over the brachial artery or directly to the probe (transducer).

Position the manometer at eye level.

Gently place the probe (transducer) over the brachial artery touching the skin at a 45 to 90 degree angle.

Turn the On–Off switch on the Doppler to the On position and adjust the volume control.

Listen for a pulsating or wavelike swooshing sound, moving the probe slightly while maintaining skin contact until the sound is detected.

Estimate the systolic pressure by listening for the sound while inflating the cuff.

Note the reading on the manometer at which the sound disappears (estimated systolic pressure).

Deflate the cuff and wait 30 seconds.

Replace the probe (transducer) as above and inflate the cuff to 30 mmHg above the estimated systolic pressure.

Deflate the cuff slowly and steadily at an approximate rate of 2 to 3 mmHg per second.

Note the readings on the manometer at which the first consecutive sounds are heard (Korotkoff I) and at which the sounds become muffled (Korotkoff IV).

Record these readings as the systolic and diastolic pressures, respectively. Note the use of a Doppler.

Normal Findings	*Abnormal Findings*
Systolic pressure 100 to 140 mmHg	Systolic pressure <100 mmHg or >140 mmHg
Diastolic pressure 60 to 90 mmHg	Diastolic pressure <60 mmHg or >90 mmHg
Difference in blood pressure between arms <10 mmHg	Difference in blood pressure between arms >10 mmHg
Difference in systolic blood pressure between sitting, lying, and standing positions <25 mmHg; difference in diastolic blood pressure between sitting, lying and standing positions <10 mmHg	Difference in systolic blood pressure between sitting, lying, and standing positions >25 mmHg; difference in diastolic blood pressure between sitting, lying and standing positions >10 mmHg (orthostatic hypotension)
	Dizziness; lightheadedness; cool, clammy skin

Geriatric Considerations

Normal Findings

Body contours	Sharpened angles; subcutaneous fat lost from face, arms and legs; fat concentrates on hips and lower abdomen
Posture	Somewhat stooped as the thoracic spine becomes more convex
Gait	Speed, balance, coordination decrease in advanced age
Height	Decreases with age because of kyphosis, flexion of knees and hips, shrinking of the vertebrae and the intervertebral discs, and presence of osteoporosis
Weight	Gradual weight gain if caloric intake remains constant and life-style becomes more sedentary
	Decreased with very old age

Pulse	Remains constant during rest, with exercise may take longer to return to baseline
	Radial artery may feel rigid and tortuous
Respirations	Remains constant during rest; with exercise may take longer to return to baseline
Blood pressure	Gradual increase in both systolic and diastolic values; tendency to develop orthostatic hypotension

Clinical Notes

Geriatric patients are less likely to develop fever but more likely to develop hypothermia than younger adults.

Obtain an accurate height. Older person's self-report may be inaccurate as he or she may be unaware of height loss.

Pediatric Considerations

Equipment

Table scale
Tape measure
Standardized growth charts for height, weight, and head circumference
Standardized blood pressure percentile graphs
Pediatric blood pressure cuff

Procedure

<36 months: measure length from the vertex of the head to the heels.

>36 months: measure standing height.

Measure head circumference around the largest circumference of the cranium over the occipital prominence, above the ears, and above the eyebrows. Repeat two more times and take the average.

Measure chest circumference over the nipple line.

Age Group	Normal Values
Newborn	Heart rate: 80 to 160 beats/minute

	Respiratory rate: 30 to 60/minute
Infants 1 to 3 months	Heart rate: 100 to 220 beats/minute
	Respiratory rate: 30/minute
Infants 3 Months to 2 Years	Heart rate: 70 to 120 beats/minute
	Respiratory rate: 25 to 30/minute
Children 2 Years to Adolescence	Heart rate: 60 to 110 beats/minute
	Respiratory rate: 20/minute
Adolescents	Heart rate: 50 to 90 beats/minute
	Respiratory rate: 16 to 20/minute

| *Normal Findings* | *Abnormal Findings* |
| Upper limits obtained with activity | Upper limits exceeded with illness or pathology |

Clinical Notes

Norms for vital signs vary with age and level of activity.
Take the apical pulse in children <2 years; count for one
full minute.

In infants, respirations are diaphragmatic and irregular;
measure for one full minute at the diaphragm.

Blood pressure can be measured by auscultation, palpation
(the point at which the radial pulse is felt upon deflation
of the cuff), or use of a Doppler instrument.

4

Nutritional Assessment

Knowledge of an individual's nutritional status is essential to the assessment of the person's general health. Nutritional status represents the balance between the nutritional and energy needs of the body for carbohydrates, proteins, fats, vitamins, and minerals, and the consumption of these nutrients. Malnutrition, or an altered nutritional status, results from either undernutrition or overnutrition (nutritional deprivation or excess), and directly impacts upon the promotion, maintenance, and restoration of an individual's health.

The total picture of an individual's nutritional status is assessed in a number of ways, including a history of nutritional patterns and health- and illness-related information, anthropometric measurements, a physical examination, and analysis of laboratory data.

The basic nutritional status and nutritional needs of each person must be assessed to identify individuals with, or at risk for, poor nutritional status. Such individuals may require further evaluation, and referral to other health care professionals and/or social services for nutrition counseling, support, and/or intervention. A complete nutritional assessment may not be necessary for each person.

HISTORY AND CURRENT STATUS QUESTIONS

Eating pattern/habits?   Number of meals per day,
                                      number of snacks per day,

usual meal times, types of food consumed, usual amounts consumed, food likes, food dislikes, eating out

Consider cultural and/or religious variations (e.g., the prohibition of pork and shellfish from the diet of Orthodox Jewish and Seventh Day Adventist individuals, and periods of fasting among Muslim and Jewish persons)

Socioeconomic/functional status?

Educational level, knowledge of basic nutrition, sufficient or insufficient finances, who shops for food, who prepares meals, adequacy of food storage and food preparation facilities (i.e., refrigerator and stove), eat alone or with others, assistance with ADLs, home meal delivery

Changes in weight?

Current weight, recent weight changes (gain or loss), date of occurrence, number of pounds, over how long a period of time, intentional or unintentional, precipitating factors, content or discontent with present weight, family history of obesity

Changes in appetite?

Date of onset, increase or decrease, over how long a period of time, particular time of day, presence of nausea, vomiting, indigestion, early satiety

Changes in taste perception?	Date of onset, duration, precipitating factors
Difficulty chewing?	Date of onset, precipitating factors or cause if known, description of pain if present, dental history (i.e. dentures, missing teeth, unfilled caries)
Difficulty swallowing?	Date of onset, duration, solids and/or liquids, precipitating factors, treatment, presence of pain and/or hoarseness
Changes in bowel habits?	Date of onset, duration, diarrhea, constipation, pain, precipitating factors, treatment
Illness, surgery, special treatments (i.e., diabetes mellitus, AIDS, chemotherapy, depression, osteoporosis)?	Date of occurrence, duration, type (including recent stress, trauma, extensive dental work), treatment
Eating disorders (i.e., anorexia nervosa, bulimia)?	Date of onset, duration, type, treatment, outcome of treatment
Nutritional counseling?	Reason, duration, frequency, by whom, type, last visit, hospitalization
Special or prescribed diet?	Date begun, duration, medical restrictions (e.g., sodium restrictions), cultural and/or religious restrictions [i.e., Kosher diet, natural or health foods, vegetarian (type)], dietary supplements, cholesterol levels if known
Food allergies/intolerances?	Date of onset, allergens, symptoms, treatment, effectiveness of relief measures
	Consider cultural variations

(e.g., prevalence of lactose intolerance among Mexican
Americans, African Americans
and Native Americans)

Medications?   Type, prescription, over the
counter, starting date, when
last taken, dose, frequency, vitamins, nutrient supplements,
appetite suppressants, illegal
drugs

Alcohol, caffeine, tobacco?   Type, amount per day, frequency, Alcoholics Anonymous

Exercise?   Type, frequency, intensity,
duration

PHYSICAL EXAMINATION

Equipment

Floor model platform scale with height measuring attach-
ment
Tape measure
Stethoscope
Sphygmomanometer and cuff
Watch with a second hand
Skinfold calipers
Tongue blade
Penlight
Paper
Pen

Procedures, Techniques, and Findings

Procedure	*Technique*
1. Note the nutritional ade-quacy of the dietary intake	Ask the patient to recall all the food and fluids consumed in the past 24 hours
	Instruct the patient to include the types, and amounts of

	foods as well as sauces and methods of preparation
	Ask the patient if this is a typical day
	Compare the reported intake to the recommendations for food consumption set forth in the food guide pyramid (see Appendix 3)
2. Obtain the patient's weight and height	Determine weight and height as described in Chapter 3, The General Physical Assessment Survey
3. Evaluate the patient's body weight	
Obtain frame size	Measure the circumference of the wrist (in centimeters); place a tape measure around the wrist where it bends (distal to the wrist bone); divide the patient's height (in centimeters) by the wrist circumference (in centimeters)
	Compare the findings to figures in Table 4–1 to determine whether frame size is small, medium, or large

TABLE 4–1
Body Frame Size Determined from Height : Wrist Circumference Ratios

	Small	Medium	Large
Men	>10.4	9.6–10.4	<9.6
Women	>11.0	10.1–11.0	<10.1

Determine the patient's ideal body weight	See recommended weight charts (see Appendix 1)
Compare the patient's actual weight to the ideal body weight (% IBW)	Use the following formula: $\%IBW = \dfrac{Actual\ weight}{Ideal\ weight} \times 100$
Determine the percentage of recent weight change (% weight change)	Use the following formula: $\% \text{ weight change} = \dfrac{Usual\ weight - Current\ weight}{Usual\ weight} \times 100$

4. Obtain additional anthropometric measures as appropriate

Measure triceps skinfold (TSF) thickness to estimate the amount of subcutaneous fat content	Explain the procedure and the purpose to the patient
	Ask the patient to expose the entire arm, including the shoulder
Consider sociocultural variations (e.g., African Americans generally have thinner TSFs than Caucasians; socioeconomic status is inversely related to the amount of body fat	Instruct the patient to stand with the nondominant arm relaxed and extended at the side (patients who are unable to stand may sit; immobilized patients should be positioned with the arm extended across the chest)
	Locate the midpoint of the upper arm by measuring the distance from the acromion process of the scapula to the olecranon process of the elbow and dividing by 2; mark the midpoint on the back of the arm (Fig. 4–1)

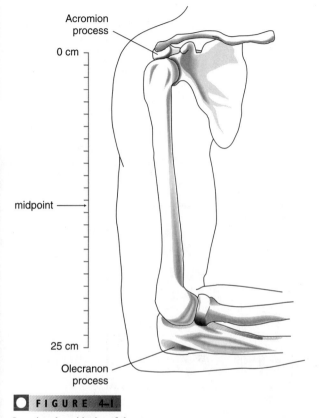

Acromion
process

0 cm

midpoint

25 cm

Olecranon
process

● FIGURE 4-1

Locating the midpoint of the upper arm.

Firmly pinch a fold of skin and
subcutaneous fat lengthwise
between the thumb and forefinger slightly above the midpoint and pull the fold away
from any underlying muscle

Place the teeth of the calipers on either side of the skinfold at the marked midpoint (Fig. 4–2)

Wait approximately 2 seconds, until the movement of the gauge stops, and note the measurement to the nearest millimeter

To improve reliability, repeat this measurement two additional times, then average the findings

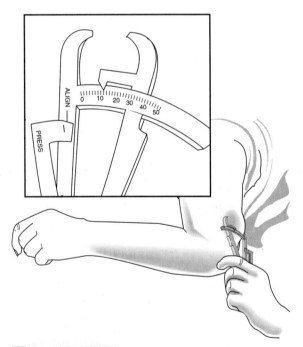

FIGURE 4–2

Use of skinfold calipers.

TABLE 4–2
Standard Anthropometric Measurements

	Male	Female
Triceps skinfold	12.5 mm	16.5 mm
Midarm circumference	29.3 cm	28.5 cm
Midarm muscle circumference	25.3 cm	23.2 cm

Record the average finding and compare to the standard measurements listed in Table 4–2

Calculate the finding as a percent of the standard measurement as follows:

$$\frac{\text{Actual measurement}}{\text{Standard measurement}} \times 100$$

Measure midarm circumference (MAC) to estimate both the fat and skeletal muscle content of the arm

Explain the procedure and the purpose to the patient

Prepare and position the patient as for the TSF measurement

Place the tape measure around the upper arm at the marked midpoint

Measure the circumference to the nearest centimeter

Record the finding and compare to the standard measurements listed in Table 4–2

Calculate the finding as a percent of the standard measurement as follows:

$$\frac{\text{Actual measurement}}{\text{Standard measurement}} \times 100$$

| Calculate the midarm muscle circumference (MAMC) to estimate the skeletal muscle mass and protein stores | Use the following formula:

MAMC (cm) =
Midarm Circumference (cm)
$- [0.314 \times$ triceps skinfold (mm)]

Record the finding and compare to the standard measurements listed in Table 4–2

Calculate the finding as a percent of the standard measurement as follows:

$$\dfrac{\text{Actual measurement}}{\text{Standard measurement}} \times 100$$ |
| 5. Note any clinical signs of malnutrition (Table 4–3) | See chapters related to specific body parts and/or systems for detailed examination techniques

Observe general mental response

Observe physical activity/energy level |

T A B L E   4–3
Manifestations of Nutritional Deficiency in Malabsorption Syndrome

Malabsorbed Nutrient	Clinical Manifestations
Protein	Weight loss, muscle wasting, alopecia, peripheral edema
Carbohydrate	Weight loss, diarrhea, flatulence, abdominal distention
Fat	Weight loss, diarrhea, steatorrhea, dermatitis

T A B L E 4–3
Manifestations of Nutritional Deficiency in Malabsorption Syndrome *Continued*

Malabsorbed Nutrient	Clinical Manifestations
Vitamin A	Epithelial keratinization, follicular hyperkeratosis, skin and mucous membrane infections
Thiamin (B_1)	Anorexia, constipation, fatigue, depression, apathy, neuritis in the legs, cardiac failure
Riboflavin (B_2)	Glossitis, cheilosis, dermatitis, photophobia
Folic acid	Macrocytic and megaloblastic anemia, glossitis, cheilosis, dermatitis
Niacin	Dermatitis, weakness, anorexia, diarrhea, apathy, depression, mental confusion
Pyridoxine	Nervous irritability, weakness, hypochromic and microcytic anemia, seborrhea-like skin lesions
Vitamin B_{12}	Pernicious anemia, glossitis, cheilosis, peripheral neuropathy, paresthesias
Vitamin D	Softening of the bones, bone deformity, bone pain, fractures, muscle weakness, tetany
Vitamin K	Bruising, bleeding, hematuria, hypoprothrombinemia, prolonged clotting time
Calcium	Positive Trousseau's and Chvostek's signs, tetany, osteoporosis, osteomalacia, bone pain, fractures, hypertension
Iron	Brittle nails, anemia, glossitis, cheilosis, stomatitis, decreaed resistance to infection
Sodium	Muscle cramps, weakness
Zinc	Dermatitis
Potassium	Muscle flaccidity, weakness, decreased tendon reflexes, cardiac dysrhythmias
Magnesium	Neuromuscular dysfunction, muscle spasms, tremors, tetany, anorexia, nausea, decreased tendon reflexes, apathy, personality changes, cardiac dysrhythmias
Phosphate	Osteomalacia
Water	Dehydration

Source: Monahon, F.D., Drake, T., Neighbors, M. Nursing Care of Adults. Philadelphia: W.B. Saunders. 1994; p. 984

Observe for edema

Observe musculoskeletal development

Inspect condition of hair

Inspect condition of skin

Inspect condition of nails

Inspect condition of lips

Inspect condition of tongue

Inspect condition of gums

Inspect condition of teeth

Inspect condition of eyes

Check tendon reflexes, balance, vibration, and position sense

Palpate the thyroid gland

Palpate the liver and spleen

6. Obtain the patient's pulse and blood pressure

Determine the pulse and blood pressure as described in Chapter 3, The General Physical Assessment Survey

7. Note laboratory values

Consider sociocultural variations (e.g., Mexican Americans tend to have higher hematocrits than Caucasians; serum cholesterol levels tend to be high in African American women and Russian Americans; American Eskimos have a high inci-

Review the patient's laboratory data to determine the following values:

Hemoglobin

Hematocrit

RBC indices

Serum electrolytes

Serum glucose

Serum lipids

Serum albumin

dence of iron deficiency
anemia)

Total protein

Urinary creatinine excretion

Serum transferrin

Serum iron

Serum ferritin

Total lymphocyte count

Total iron binding capacity

Vitamin levels

Mineral levels

	Normal Findings	*Abnormal Findings*
Nutritional intake	Food and fluid consumption is adequate and well balanced according to established guidelines	Food and fluid consumption is inadequate or excessive according to established guidelines
Weight	Weight within desired range for sex, age, and height Weight within 10% of IBW Weight change less than 10% in a 6-month period	Underweight: 10 to 15% below IBW (85 to 90% IBW) Emaciated (undernutrition): >15% below IBW (<85% IBW) Overweight: 10 to 20% above IBW (110 to 120% IBW) Obesity (overnutrition): >20% above IBW (>120% IBW)

		Unintentional weight change >10% in a 6-month period
Triceps skinfold (TSF)	Values within 10% of standard reference	Values >10% below standard reference (undernutrition, caloric deprivation)
		Values >10% above standard reference (overnutrition, excess caloric intake)
Midarm circumference (MAC)	Values within 10% of standard reference	Values >10% below the standard reference (undernutrition)
Midarm muscle circumference (MAMC)	Values within 10% of standard reference	Values >10% below the standard reference (undernutrition)
Clinical signs		
General mental response	Alert, responsive, good attention span	Apathetic, inattentive, listless, confused, disoriented, irritable
Physical activity level	Energetic, vigorous, sleeps well	Tired, fatigued, lethargic, weak, sleep disturbances
Edema	Absence of peripheral edema and ascites	Edema of feet, ankles, and/or legs, ascites

Muskuloskeletal development	Firm, developed muscles, good muscle tone, good posture, absence of skeletal deformities	Poorly developed muscles, flaccidity, muscle wasting, muscle weakness, poor posture, bowed legs, bone tenderness
Hair	Shiny hair, firmly rooted	Thin, dull, dry, brittle hair, falls out easily, decreased pigment
Skin	Skin smooth, slightly moist, color good, absence of lesions	Skin pale, cyanosis, jaundice, rough, dry, bumpy, scaly, cracked, poor turgor, striae, dark circles under the eyes, echymosis, petechiae, intolerance to cold
Nails	Nails firm, pink, smooth	Nails soft, pale, spoon shaped, ridged
Lips	Lips smooth, moist, pink	Lips dry, chapped, cracked, swollen, lesions at corners of mouth
Tongue	Tongue dark pink, rough surface with papillae present, absence of lesions	Tongue dark red or purple, swollen, smooth surface, hypertrophy of papillae, irritated, lesions

Gums	Gums pink, firm, absence of bleeding and swelling, absence of lesions	Gums red, swollen, bleeding, spongy, receding, lesions
Teeth	Teeth free of caries, discoloration and pain	Teeth loose, missing, unfilled caries, mottling, pain
Eyes	Eyes clear, bright	Eyes dry, red, dull, conjunctiva pale, Bitot's spots
Neurological signs	Tendon reflexes within normal limits, balance, vibration, and position sense present Absence of paresthesias	Tendon reflexes, balance, vibration and position sense decreased Paresthesias present
Thyroid gland	Thyroid gland size within normal limits, symmetrical	Thyroid enlarged, asymmetrical
Liver and spleen	Liver and spleen size with normal limits, absence of tenderness	Liver and spleen enlarged, tenderness
Pulse and blood pressure	Pulse and blood pressure within normal range for age	Arrythmias, hypertension, hypotension
Laboratory values	Laboratory values within normal range (see Appendix 4)	Laboratory values above or below normal range

Geriatric Considerations

History and Physical Examination

Use a level 1 screen (see Fig. 4–3) to aid in identifying older individuals who require further evaluation or who would likely benefit from a referral to an appropriate health care or social service professional.

Normal Findings

Edentulous	Poor-fitting dentures may decrease nutrition intake, limit variety in diet, and contribute to difficulty swallowing
Height decreases with age secondary to changes in intravertebral discs, vertebra, and posture	Self-reporting of height may be incorrect, leading to inaccurate body mass index
Saliva decreases, gastric motility and peristaltic activity slows	A feeling of fullness and constipation may discourage adequate nutritional intake

Clinical Notes

Multiple medications, antacids, and laxatives can interfere with nutrient absorption; a complete drug history is a necessary part of an older adult's nutritional assessment. Limiting fluid intake is often a method older adults utilize to control incontinence; assess daily fluid pattern for adequate intake.

Pediatric Considerations

Refer to Table 4–4 for assessment of nutritional status, factors placing children at risk, use of vitamins, and general nutritional guidelines by age.

Level I Screen

Name: **Date:**

Body Weight

Measure height to the nearest inch and weight to the nearest pound. Record the values below and mark them on the Body Mass Index (BMI) scale to the right. Then use a straight edge (ruler) to connect the two points and circle the spot where this straight line crosses the center line (body mass index). Record the number below.

Healthy older adults should have a BMI between 24 and 27.

Height: (in): _____
Weight (lbs): _____
Body Mass Index: _____
(number from center column)

Check any boxes that are true for the individual:

❑ Has lost or gained 10 pounds (or more) in the past 6 months.

❑ Body mass index <24

❑ Body mass index >27

For the remaining sections, please ask the individual which of the statements (if any) is true for him or her and place a check by each that applies.

Eating Habits

❑ Does not have enough food to eat each day

❑ Usually eats alone

❑ Does not eat anything on one or more days each month

❑ Has poor appetite

❑ Is on a special diet

❑ Eats vegetables two or fewer times daily

❑ Eats milk or milk products once or not at all daily

❑ Eats fruit or drinks fruit juice once or not at all daily

❑ Eats breads, cereals, pasta, rice, or other grains five or fewer times daily

● **FIGURE 4-3**

Level 1 screen.

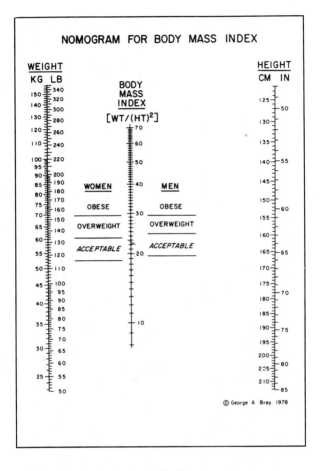

NOMOGRAM FOR BODY MASS INDEX

© George A Bray 1978

❏ Has difficulty chewing or swallowing

❏ Has more than one alcoholic drink per day (if woman) more than two drinks per day (if man)

❏ Has pain in mouth, teeth, or gums

FIGURE 4-3 *Continued*

Level 1 screen.

Illustration continued on following page

A physician should be contacted if the individual has gained or lost 10 pounds unexpectedly or without intending to during the past 6 months. A physician should also be notified if the individual's body mass index is above 27 or below 24.

Living Environment

❑ Lives on an income of less than $6000 per year (per individual in the household)

❑ Lives alone

❑ Is housebound

❑ Is concerned about home security

❑ Lives in a home with inadequate heating or cooling

❑ Does not have a stove and/or refrigerator

❑ Is unable or prefers not to spend money on food (<$25–30 per person spent on food each week)

Functional Status

Usually or always needs assistance with (check each that apply):

❑ Bathing

❑ Dressing

❑ Grooming

❑ Toileting

❑ Eating

❑ Walking or moving about

❑ Traveling (outside the home)

❑ Preparing food

❑ Shopping for food or other necessities

If you have checked one or more statements on this screen, the individual you have interviewed may be at risk for poor nutritional status. Please refer this individual to the appropriate health care or social service professional in your area. For example, a dietitian should be contacted for problems with selecting, preparing, or eating a healthy diet, or a dentist if the individual experiences pain or difficulty when chewing or swallowing. Those individuals whose income, lifestyle, or functional status may endanger their nutritional and overall health should be referred to available community services: home-delivered meals, congregate meal programs, transportation services, couseling services (alcohol abuse, depression, bereavement, etc.), home health care agencies, day care programs, etc.

Please repeat this screen at least once a year—sooner if the individual has a major change in his or her health, income, immediate family (e.g., spouse dies), or functional status.

● **FIGURE 4–3** *Continued*

TABLE 4–4
Pediatric Nutrition

Assessing Nutritional Status

Essentially the same assessment as for the adult, with the exception of reviewing growth charts for percentile ranking and appropriate curve

Factors Placing Children at Risk

Poverty
Parental neglect
Chronic illness
Weight-reduction diets
Teenage pregnancy
Fad diets, especially in the adolescent population
Substance abuse

Infancy

Breastfeeding:
  Recommended to 1 year of age
  May experience a benign jaundice between 2 and 6 weeks
  May bottle supplement after well established on the breast, usually after 2 weeks
  Expressed breast milk may be kept at room temperature for 30 minutes; refrigerated for 48 hours; frozen for 3 months in a separate door freezer; or frozen for 6 months in a deep freezer (0°F)
  Water supplements are neither recommended nor necessary in infancy until solid foods are added to the diet

Formula Feeding:
  Recommended to 1 year of age
  Available in "ready to feed," concentrate, or powder form
  Recommended to use formula with iron added at 12 mg/liter
  (*Note:* There is no evidence to support the idea that formula with iron causes constipation, therefore the formula with iron should be continued and constipation, if it develops, should be treated as a separate issue.)
  A cow's milk protein-based formula is recommended for all infants
  Infants with a lactose intolerance may use a lactose-free formula and infants with a *true* cow's milk allergy may use a soy protein-based formula
  Infant's with malabsorption syndromes may use a hydrolyzed protein formula

Table continued on following page

T A B L E   4–4
Pediatric Nutrition *(Continued)*

Supplemental Feedings:

  Solid food should be introduced as single-ingredient foods rather than in combined forms like "mixed dinners"

  Solid foods should be introduced one at a time for 5 to 7 days in order to more easily identify the causative agent of food reactions

  Do *not* add cereal or any other solid foods to a bottle: this deprives the child of necessary developmental experience

  Solid food should be added to the diet when the infant is able to sit with support and has good neuromuscular control; this is usually between 4 and 6 months

  The infant ready to eat solid food will indicate desire by opening the mouth and leaning forward; readiness is influenced by growth, development, and activity level

  The sequence in which foods are introduced is *not* critical, although a single-grain, iron-fortified cereal like rice cereal is usually recommended as the first solid food

  Either commercially prepared pureed foods or table foods that have been pureed or chopped are appropriate solids in infancy

  Juice may be introduced at the same time fruits are added to the diet

Childhood (1–12 years)

"RDA" (recommended dietary allowances) are published for children by the Food and Nutrition Board, National Academy of Sciences

Twenty-four-hour caloric intake should comprise:

  Below 2 years:
  Protein: 10–15%
  Fat: 25–30%
  Carbohydrate: 50–60%

  Over 2 years:
  Protein: 25–30%
  Fat: 10–15%
  Carbohydrate: 50–60%

Maintenance calories and 24-hour fluid volume is calculated as follows:

  ADD for *each* kg of body weight:
      100 for *each* of the first 10 kg
       50 for *each* of the next 10 kg
    ___ 20 for *each* kg above the first 20 kg
    TOTAL = calories and/or fluid volume/24 hours

Childhood is the period when dietary patterns and habits are usually set for life

Foods from the basic food groups, below, need *only* be eaten every 2 to 3 days
  Dairy
  Meat, fish, poultry, eggs, nuts, legumes
  Vegetables
  Fruits
  Cereal, rice, pasta, bread

Neither skim nor low fat milk (1%, 2%) should be substituted for whole milk until after 2 years of age
Some helpful guidelines include:
  Milk at 2 to 3 cups per day
  Eggs at 3 to 4 times per week
  Breakfast cereals with a low sugar content
  Finger foods of vegetables and fruit
  Discourage "snacking" in front of the television
  Establish a family eating time
  Caution early against alcohol, smoking, caffeine, and "junk" foods

Adolescence

Independence, peer pressure, and busy schedules lead to altered dietary habits
Consider increased caloric needs because of high-energy activities like sports
Observe for skipping meals, snacking, fast food intake, dieting
Observe for obesity, iron-deficiency anemia, dental caries, and eating disorders
Special diets (e.g., vegetarian) may lead to special deficiencies if not well planned

Vitamins and Minerals

Vitamins are added to all commercially prepared formulas; supplements are *not* needed in infancy
Multivitamin supplements are only needed for the breastfed infant if the mother is malnourished
Vitamin K may be needed if an infant's skin is deeply pigmented and there is limited exposure to sunlight
Fluoride supplements are recommended, beginning at 6 months of age, to prevent dental caries or when the community water supply has less than 0.3 ppm of fluoride; remember, even in communities where the water is fluorinated, ready-to-food formula deprives the infant of that fluoride
Iron must be added to the diet at 6 months and is usually supplied by iron-fortified formula and solid foods

Committee on Nutrition: Pediatric Nutrition Handbook, 3rd ed., American Academy of Pediatrics, Elk Grove, IL, 1993.

5

Mental Status Assessment

The assessment of an individual's mental status focuses on cognitive functioning and the emotional status of the patient. The examination includes a description of the patient's general appearance, level of consciousness, orientation, communication and language functioning, mood, memory, ability to concentrate, judgment, general intellectual ability, and thought processes. Much of this information can be obtained from general interaction with the patient during the health history interview and physical examination from observation and conversation. Knowledge and awareness of the patient's age, educational background, sociocultural factors, and communication barriers (such as English as a second language and aphasia) are essential to the accurate and valid assessment of mental status.

HISTORY AND CURRENT STATUS QUESTIONS

Head injury?

Description, date of occurrence, symptoms, residual effects

Stroke (CVA)?	Date of occurrence, symptoms, treatment, residual effects
Headaches?	Location, description of pain, frequency, constant or recurrent, time of onset, duration, precipitating factors, associated factors, relief measures utilized, effectiveness of relief measures
Seizures?	Onset, cause if known, type, aura, loss of consciousness, incontinence, time of last seizure, treatment
Changes in memory?	Onset, long-term memory, short-term memory, loss of memory
Changes in speech?	Onset, type, cause if known, treatment
Mood?	Onset, duration, intensity, steady, changing, swings
Mental health counseling?	Duration, frequency, reason, by whom, type, last visit, hospitalization
Alcoholism?	Date of onset, duration, treatment, Alcoholics Anonymous
Medications?	Type (sedatives, hypnotics, antianxiety, antidepressant, antipsychotic, analgesics, stimulants), date first used, frequency, duration, effectiveness
	Use of illegal drugs
Educational background?	Last grade completed, high school, college

PHYSICAL EXAMINATION

Equipment

Pencil
Paper
Reading material

Procedures, Techniques, and Findings

Procedure	*Technique*
1. Note the patient's general appearance, including personal hygiene and dress, manner and affect, facial expressions, posture, and motor activity	See Chapter 3, General Physical Assessment Survey
Consider sociocultural factors, such as variations in manner of dress	
2. Note the level of consciousness	
Check arousability	Observe whether the patient is fully awake
	If the patient is asleep or unconscious, call the patient by name in an increasingly loud voice
	If there is no response, continue to increase the stimulus by touching the arm, gently shaking the shoulder, or producing a painful stimulus as necessary until a response is elicited
	Apply a painful stimulus by pressing on the base of the thumb nailbed

	Terminate the painful stimulus as soon as a response is noted
Check motor responses	Ask the patient to open his or her eyes or squeeze your hand
	Observe the motor response to a painful stimulus if necessary
3. Note orientation	Determine the patient's orientation to time, place, and person during the course of the interview and conversation
Check awareness of time	If necessary, ask the patient to state the correct date, including the day, month, and year
Check awareness of place	If necessary, ask the patient to state the name of the hospital or health care facility, or home address
Check awareness of person	If necessary, ask the patient to state his or her full name, age, or the name of a significant other who is present
Check awareness of situation	If necessary, ask the patient to describe what has occurred relative to the present illness

4. Note communication and language function

Consider sociocultural variables such as English as a second language

Check ability to speak	Observe clarity, quality, rate, inflection and quantity of speech
	Observe whether speech is spontaneous or hesitant

Observe whether patient uses full sentences, phrases, and appropriate words

Observe whether speech pattern is organized

Ask the patient to repeat one or two words or phrases

Check ability to understand

Determine the patient's ability to understand questions and instructions during the course of the interview and conversation

If necessary, ask the patient to follow simple commands such as to stick out his or her tongue or to touch his or her ear

If necessary, point to at least five familiar objects and ask the patient to identify them by name

If necessary, name objects and ask the patient to point to them

Check ability to write

Ask the patient to write his or her name and a simple sentence

Check ability to read

Ask the patient to read a simple sentence aloud

5. Note mood

Observe affect throughout the course of the interview and conversation

Ask the patient how he or she is feeling

	Ask the patient what his or her future plans are
	If necessary, ask the patient if he or she ever thinks about hurting himself or herself, or that life is no longer worth living

6. Note memory

Test remote (long-term) memory	Ask the patient questions about past events that can be validated, such as dates of anniversaries or historical events
Test recent (short-term) memory	Ask the patient to recall a mutually known event that occurred earlier in the day or within the previous 24 hours
Test immediate (recall) memory	Give the patient two or three common objects to remember; ask the patient to list them 5 to 10 minutes later

7. Note ability to concentrate — Observe the patient's ability to focus and attend to conversation and tasks

Test attention span	Ask the patient to repeat a series of five or six digits forward and then backward

< and / or >

Ask the patient to subtract 7 from 100, then to continue subtracting 7 from each answer (stop after 5 subtractions)

< and / or >

Ask the patient to spell the word WORLD backward

Test abstract thinking	Ask the patient to explain a proverb such as "A stitch in time saves nine," or "The early bird catches the worm"
Consider sociocultural variables (e.g., the interpretation of certain proverbs may be culturally dependent)	Ask the patient to explain why similar items are alike (e.g., a pear and a banana)
8. Note judgment	Ask the patient questions such as "What would you do if there was a fire in the wastebasket?"
9. Note intellectual ability	
Test general knowledge	Ask the patient general knowledge questions such as "Who is the president of the United States?", "What is the capital of France?", "What are the four seasons of the year?", and "What are the names of two oceans?"
Test vocabulary	Observe the patient's use of vocabulary during the course of conversation
Consider sociocultural variables such as English as a second language	Ask the patient to define vocabulary words, beginning with the least difficult and progressing to the most difficult words
Test calculation ability	Ask the patient to mentally perform simple arithmetic problems involving the four basic operations (addition, subtraction, multiplication, and division)
	Ask the patient to solve a simple problem, such as "How

much change will you receive from $1.00 after purchasing two items that cost $.30 each?"

10. Note thought process and content

Observe verbal and nonverbal communication for thought process and content during the course of conversation

If necessary ask the patient questions to gain further insight into abnormalities of content and/or perceptions

	Normal Findings	*Abnormal Findings*
General Appearance	See Chapter 3, General Physical Assessment Survey	
Level of Consciousness		
Arousability	Awake, alert, readily aroused	Not fully alert, drowsy, lethargic, stuporous, comatose
	Responsive to minimal external stimuli	Difficult to arouse
Motor response	Follows commands	Reduced or slowed response
	Responds appropriately and quickly	Responds only to shaking or painful stimulation, purposeful or nonpurposeful responses
		No motor response to painful stimuli
Orientation	Oriented and aware of time, place, and person	Disoriented, unaware of time, place, and/or person

Communication
and language
function

Ability to speak

Speech is clear, smooth, understandable, moderately paced, spontaneous and effortless

Speech is unclear, difficult to understand, fast, slow, loud, soft, hesitant, monotone, slurred

Normal volume, pitch, quantity

Speaks minimally, excessively, only in response to questions

Uses full sentences, appropriate and relevant choice of words

Uses incomplete sentences, inappropriate choice of words, misuse of words

Organized speech patterns

Disorganized speech patterns

Correctly repeats words and phrases

Unable to repeat words and phrases, substitutes words, creates words

Ability to understand

Understands questions and responds appropriately and readily

Unable to respond to questions appropriately

Responds slowly

Follows instructions and correctly performs commands

Unable to follow instructions and perform commands

Correctly identifies and names familiar objects

Unable to identify familiar objects by name, identifies function

	Correctly points out selected objects	Unable to point out selected objects
Ability to write	Correctly writes his or her name and a simple sentence	Unable to write his or her name or sentence
Ability to read	Correctly reads a sentence aloud	Unable to read
Mood	Mood and affect are appropriate to situation and discussion	Flat, inappropriate affect
	Even mood and affect	Euphoria, hopelessness, depression, indifference, withdrawn, extreme anger, hostility, severe anxiety
		Emotional lability
		Use of drugs and/or alcohol
Memory		
Remote memory	Recalls remote events readily and accurately	Unable to recall remote events
		Makes up answers
Recent memory	Recalls events of the day clearly	Unable to recall events of the day
Immediate memory	Repeats stated objects completely and accurately	Unable to recall stated objects
Concentration	Remains focused, completes thoughts and activities	Easily distracted, fidgets
Attention span	Repeats a series of digits forward and backward, repeat-	Unable to repeat a series of digits, repeatedly subtract

	edly subtracts the number 7 from 100, and spells WORLD backward, effortlessly, quickly and accurately	7 from 100, and/or spell WORLD. backward
Abstract thinking	Interprets and explains proverb accurately	Unable to explain proverb and/or to identify similarities
	Identifies and explains similarities accurately	
Judgment	Accurately interprets the situation and draws logical conclusions	Unable to interpret the situation and draw logical conclusions
	Expresses thoughts clearly	
Intellectual ability		
General knowledge	Correctly answers general knowledge questions	Unable to answer questions
Vocabulary	Vocabulary use is appropriate for age, educational level, and cultural background	Inappropriate use of vocabulary
	Able to define selected words	Unable to define selected words
Calculation ability	Completes mental calculations with few errors	Unable to perform mental calculations accurately
	Able to solve problem correctly	Unable to solve problem
Thought process and content	Thoughts expressed are clear,	Thoughts expressed are inco-

complete, organized, logical, connected, relevant, and flow freely	herent, illogical, incomplete, irrelevant, and confusing Flight of ideas
Content and perceptions are based in reality	Content and/or perceptions are not reality based
	Obsession, phobia, delusions, hallucinations

Clinical Notes

The Glasgow Coma Scale may be used as an additional objective assessment tool to evaluate level of consciousness (see Appendix 5). The Mini Mental State Examination may be used as a quick additional assessment tool to evaluate mental status (Table 5–1).

Geriatric Considerations

Hearing and vision loss can cause an inaccurate assessment of orientation. Be sure hearing aids and glasses are in place.

Older adults have more potential for loss. Grief and depression can affect mental status.

Response to questions slows with age. Allow adequate response time.

Confusion is not a normal aging change. If confusion is present, determine whether symptoms have developed rapidly or progressed gradually over time.

Pediatric Considerations

History

Is there age appropriate interaction:

Newborn:	Bonding with primary caretaker?
Infant:	Recognizes strangers, demonstrates stranger anxiety?
Toddler:	Parallel play?

TABLE 5-1
Mini-Mental State Examination

Patient _____ Examiner _____ Date _____

Maximum Score	Score	
		ORIENTATION
5	( )	What is the (year) (season) (date) (day) (month)?
5	( )	Where are we: (state) (county) (town) (hospital) (floor).
		REGISTRATION
3	( )	Name 3 objects: 1 second to say each. Then ask the patient all 3 after you have said them. Give 1 point for each correct answer. Then repeat them until he learns all 3. Count trials and record. Trials _____
		ATTENTION AND CALCULATION
5	( )	Serial 7's. 1 point for each correct. Stop after 5 answers. Alternatively spell "world" backwards.
		RECALL
3	( )	Ask for the 3 objects repeated above. Give 1 point for each correct.
		LANGUAGE
9	( )	Name a pencil, and watch (2 points)
		Repeat the following "No ifs, ands, or buts." (1 point)
		Follow a 3-stage command:
		"Take a paper in your right hand, fold it in half, and put it on the floor." (3 points)
		Read and obey the following:
		CLOSE YOUR EYES (1 point)
		Write a sentence (1 point)
		Copy design (1 point)
	Total score	
		ASSESS level of consciousness along a continuum

Alert   Drowsy   Stupor   Coma

110

ORIENTATION

(1) Ask for the date. Then ask specifically for parts omitted, e.g., "Can you also tell me what season it is?" One point for each correct.

(2) Ask in turn "Can you tell me the name of this hospital?" (town, county, etc.). One point for each correct.

REGISTRATION

Ask the patient if you may test his memory. Then say the names of 3 unrelated objects, clearly and slowly, about one second for each. After you have said all 3, ask him to repeat them. This first repetition determines his score (0–3) but keep saying them until he can repeat all 3, up to 6 trials. If he does not eventually learn all 3, recall cannot be meaningfully tested.

ATTENTION AND CALCULATION

Ask the patient to begin with 100 and count backwards by 7. Stop after 5 subtractions (93, 86, 79, 72, 65). Score the total number of correct answers.

If the patient cannot or will not perform this task, ask him to spell the word "world" backwards. The score is the number of letters in correct order. E.g/ dlrow = 5, dlorw = 3.

RECALL

Ask the patient if he can recall the 3 words you previously asked him to remember. Score 0–3.

LANGUAGE

Naming: Show the patient a wrist watch and ask him what it is. Repeat for pencil. Score 0–2.

Repetition: Ask the patient to repeat the sentence after you. Allow only one trial. Score 0 or 1.

3-Stage command: Give the patient a piece of plain blank paper and repeat the command. Score 1 point for each part correctly executed.

Reading: On a blank piece of paper print the sentence "Close your eyes," in letters large enough for the patient to see clearly. Ask him to read it and do what it says. Score 1 point only if he actually closes his eyes.

Writing: Give the patient a blank piece of paper and ask him to write a sentence for you. Do not dictate a sentence, it is to be written spontaneously. It must contain a subject and verb and be sensible. Correct grammar and punctuation are not necessary.

Copying: On a clean piece of paper, draw intersecting pentagons, each side about 1 in., and ask him to copy it exactly as is is. All 10 angles must be present and 2 must intersect to score 1 point. Tremor and rotation are ignored.

Estimate the patient's level of sensorium along a continuum, from alert to coma on the left to coma on the right.

(From Folstein MF, Folstein SE, McHugh PR: Mini-mental state. J Psychiatric Res 12:189–198, 1975, Elsevier Science Ltd, Oxford, England. Reprinted with permission.)

Preschool: Cooperative play?
School-age: Group activities?
Adolescent: Dating, interest in the opposite sex?
    Maternal substance abuse during pregnancy?
    Any developmental delay?
    Any chronic illness affecting socialization and/or school
      attendance?
    Recent emotional trauma, conflicts at home?

Physical Examination

The Denver Developmental Testing Kit or other acceptable
tool is used for evaluating developmental milestones.

Normal Findings	Common Variations	Abnormal Findings
Newborn		
Lusty cry	One fussy period that occurs at approximately the same time each 24 hours; self-limiting in nature	Weak cry High-pitched cry
	Colic; frequent crying in otherwise normal baby	
Infant and Child		
		Autism: little or no interaction with others; appears to be responding to inner stimuli; normal IQ
		Attention deficit disorder: impulsive, short attention span that interferes with learning

Adolescent

| Testing limits | Experimenting with substance abuse | Addiction |
| | Experimenting with sexual activity | Promiscuity |

6

Assessment of the Skin, Hair, and Nails

HISTORY AND CURRENT STATUS QUESTIONS

Sun exposure?	Amount, frequency, time of day, use of protective clothing or lotion, SPF#
Change in skin color, texture, or moisture?	Type of change, date first discovered, constant or intermittent, frequency of occurrence, associated symptoms, precipitating or associated factors, remedies employed and their effectiveness
Change in hair texture, amount, or distribution?	
Change in nails such as color, splitting, or breaking?	
Bruising?	Areas of body affected, size of bruises, date first noted, pattern of occurrence, precipitating or aggravating factors
Change in mole?	Type of change, date first noticed
Rashes or lesions?	Location, appearance, date first noticed, precipitating or ag-

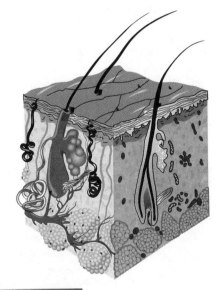

FIGURE 6-1

Basic anatomy of the skin.

	gravating factors, type and effect of self-treatment measures used
Lumps?	Location, size, consistency, mobility, date first noticed, change since discovery
Previous skin disease?	Type, date of occurrence, treatment, residual effects
Skin care behaviors?	Patterns of bathing, type of soap, cosmetics or other hygienic products used, frequency of their use
Exposure to environmental or occupational irritants/toxins?	Type (poisonous plants, irritant chemicals) time and duration of exposure

PHYSICAL EXAMINATION

Equipment

Lighting, preferably natural, strong, direct

Procedures, Techniques, and Findings

Clinical Note

Begin assessment of the skin with exposed areas such as the face, hands and arms. Assess other skin areas as the other body regions are examined.

Procedure	*Technique*
1. Inspect and palpate the skin	Expose area and clean if needed
	Use good light, natural if possible, since artificial light can distort colors and mask jaundice
Note general color as well as local, patchy variations and vascularity	Look for pallor in nail beds, lips, oral mucous membranes, and palpebral conjunctiva
	Check lips, buccal mucosa, and tongue for central cyanosis
	Check nail beds and skin of the arms and legs for peripheral cyanosis or pallor
	Look for jaundice in bulbar conjunctiva, lips, hard palate, and skin
Note temperature	Use back of hand to check general skin temperature as well as that of any reddened areas; compare bilaterally
Note moisture and texture	Use pads of the fingers

Note mobility and turgor	Pinch and lift a fold of skin over the sternum or the clavicle. Assess ease of movement and speed with which it returns to original position
Note lesions	Identify location, distribution, elevation (flat or raised), arrangement, type, color, size, mobility, and type of exudate, if any (Table 6–1)
Check for edema	Press thumb firmly over bony area of ankle, tibia, and coccyx
	Note depth and duration of any resultant indentation

2. Inspect and palpate the hair, noting quantity, distribution, color, and texture   Ask patient to remove wig or hairpiece

3. Inspect scalp   Part hair in several places; look for lesions and/or parasites

4. Inspect and palpate fingernails and toenails, noting color, shape, contour, surface smoothness, uniformity of thickness, and lesions

	Normal Findings	*Abnormal Findings*
Skin		
Color		
General	Pink tones in light-skinned persons; light to dark brown or olive in dark-skinned persons	Flushing, pallor (seen as loss of red tones in dark skin), cyanosis (seen as ash gray in dark skin), yellowing (Table 6–2).

T A B L E   6–1
Description of Skin Lesions

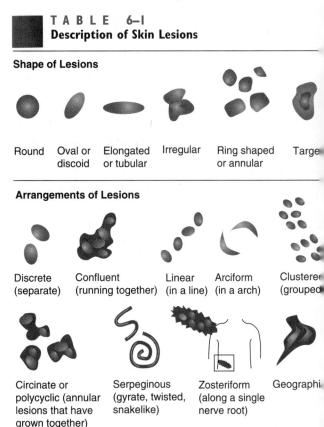

Shape of Lesions

Round | Oval or discoid | Elongated or tubular | Irregular | Ring shaped or annular | Targe

Arrangements of Lesions

Discrete (separate) | Confluent (running together) | Linear (in a line) | Arciform (in a arch) | Clustered (grouped

Circinate or polycyclic (annular lesions that have grown together) | Serpeginous (gyrate, twisted, snakelike) | Zosteriform (along a single nerve root) | Geographi

Distribution of Lesions

Regional - limited to one area of the body, eg., soles of the feet, chest, or hands
Generalized - widespread over many areas of the skin
Circumscribed - sharply limited to a specific area by a distinct borde
Scattered - "here and there" on various areas of the skin
Symmetric - same size and shape on both sides of the body
Exposed areas - areas open to the environment
Pressure sites - areas of increased pressure
Intertriginous areas - areas where skin surfaces touch

Common Variations and Abnormalities in Skin Color

Color Variation	Affected Area(s)	Common Cause(s)
Pallor	Skin, hair, eyes	Albinism
	Patchy spots on white on symmetrical and often exposed areas	Vitiligo
	Marked in face, conjunctiva, and nail beds	Syncope, shock, anemia; possible normal variation
	Edematous body areas	Nephrotic syndrome
Erythema	Face, upper chest, area of inflammation or areas exposed to cold	Blushing, fever, alcohol intake, local inflammation, exposure to cold
	Face and upper torso	CO_2 poisoning
Reddish-blue tone	Face, oral mucosa, conjunctiva, hands, feet	Polycythemia
Cyanosis (blue)	Lips, buccal mucosa, tongue, nails	Anxiety, cold exposure
		Heart, lung or blood disorder
Yellow	Skin, especially exposed areas	Chronic uremia
Jaundice	Conjunctiva, other mucous membranes, skin	Liver disease
		RBC hemolysis
Carotinemia	Palms, soles, face	Excessive intake of carotene-rich vegetables and fruits; diabetes mellitus; myxedema
Brown	"Bronze" skin, especially exposed areas, pressure sites, nipples, genitalia, palmar creases	Addison's disease (hyposecretion of the adrenal cortex)
	Face, nipples, vulva	Pregnancy

Local variations	Suntan in white-skinned persons; light lips, palms, nail beds, soles, blue-black discoloration over the sacral area, and freckle-like areas on nail beds and sclera in dark-skinned persons	Areas of increased or decreased pigmentation, erythema, ecchymosis, petechiae, purpura
Lesions	Freckles, scars, striae	Tracks, varicosities, nodules, papules, fissures, scaling, etc. (Fig. 6–2).
Temperature	Warm or cool	Hot or cold
Moisture	Dry	Excessively dry, damp, sweaty, oily
Texture	Smooth, even, soft	Rough, thick, uneven

🔘 FIGURE 6-2

Basic types of skin lesions.
  A, Macule: flat lesion characterized by a change in skin color.

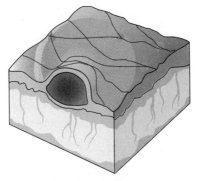

B, Papule: raised lesion < 1 cm in diameter.

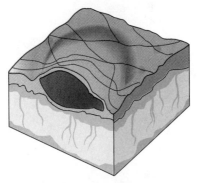

C, Plaque: raised lesion > 1 cm in diameter.

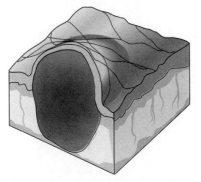

D, Nodule: raised solid mass deeper than a papule or a plaque.
Illustration continued on following page

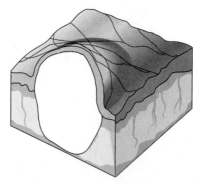

E, Cyst: mass filled with liquid or semisolid expressible material.

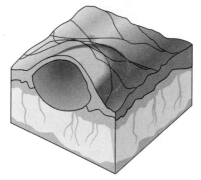

F, Pustule: cavity filled with pus that may be infectious or sterile.

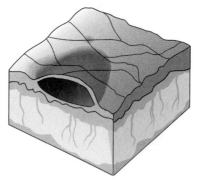

G, Wheal: transient, irregular elevation of the skin due to edema (a hive).

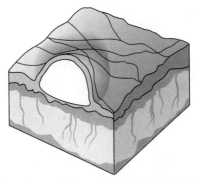

H, Vesicle: cavity containing serous fluid (a blister) of ≤ 0.5 cm.

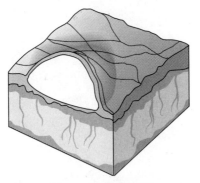

I, Bulla: cavity containing serous fluid > 0.5 cm.

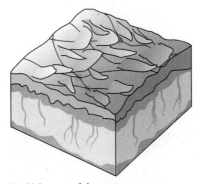

J, Scales: dry thick areas of the stratum corneum.

Illustration continued on following page

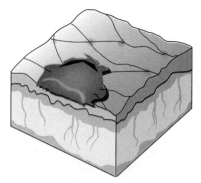

K, Crust: dried blood, serum, or pus residue.

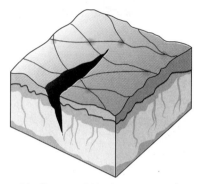

L, Fissures: thin, linear cracks in the epidermis.

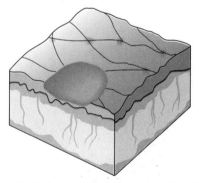

M, Erosion: shallow, scraped-out lesion in the epidermis.

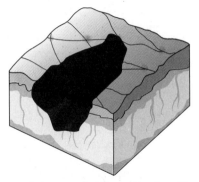

N, Ulcer: open lesion extending deeper than the epidermis.

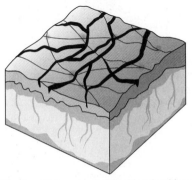

O, Lichenification: thickened areas of epidermis with prominent skin markings.

Turgor	Pinched up skinfold returns immediately to normal position	Pinched up skinfold remains tented for ≥ 5 seconds
Edema	Absent	Mild to deep pitting of skin and underlying tissue 1+ mild (2 mm pit) 2+ (4 mm pit) 3+ (6 mm pit) 4+ deep (8 mm pit)
Hair	Varied color and distribution; fine to	Patchy or sudden hair loss, brittle

	coarse texture	texture, absence of hair on the lower limbs, hirsutism
Nails	Clean, curved hard nail, smooth firm pink to light-brown nail bed; pink nail with speckled pigmentation in dark-skinned individuals; angle between nail and base 160 degrees	Dirty, jagged, soft, brittle, spooned, clubbed, or flattened nail; horizontal lines in the nail; swollen, reddened, pale, or cyanotic nail bed; splinter hemorrhages in nail bed (Table 6–3)

T A B L E   6–3
Common Variations and Abnormalities of the Nails

Variation/Abnormality	Description and Significance
Curved nails 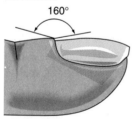	Nails have a convex curve but the angle between the nail and its base is normal Normal variation of no clinical significance
Spoon nails 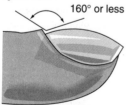	Nails are thin and have a concave curve due to the upward tilt of the edges Sometimes associated with anemia

T A B L E 6–3
Common Variations and Abnormalities
of the Nails *(Continued)*

Early clubbing

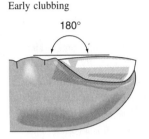

Angle between the nail and its base is straight (180 degrees)
Base is springy on palpation

Late clubbing

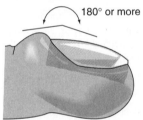

Angle between the nail and its base is greater than 180 degrees because of elevation of the proximal edge of the nail
Base is swollen and springy on palpation
Tip of finger appears rounder and wider than normal

Splinter hemorrhages

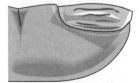

Red-brown longitudinal streaks in the nail bed
Occur in subacute bacterial endocarditis (bacterial infection of the inner lining of the heart) but also occur in other disorders, following trauma, or for no apparent reason

Beau's lines

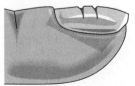

Horizontal indentation or furrow due to impaired nail formation
May be due to acute systemic illness or local trauma

Clinical Note

Melanin pigment in lips may give a false impression of cyanosis

Geriatric Considerations

	Normal Findings
Skin	Folds and sags progressing to paper-thin, dry, and wrinkled
	Senile purpura from minor trauma due to vascular fragility
	Yellow and deeply furrowed in sun-exposed areas
	Turgor decreased
	Veins more prominent
Hair	Thin, fine, gray or white, male pattern baldness in genetically prone men
	Nasal orifice, ear, and eyebrow hair coarse and thick
	Decreased pubic and axillary hair
Nails	Dull, sometimes yellowed, with longitudinal ridges; may be brittle or have peeling surface

Common Skin Lesions

Seborrheic keratoses:	Brown, greasy, warty, "stuck on" lesions found on trunk, face, hands, and arms
Cherry angiomas:	Bright red or purple, flat or raised lesions on trunk and extremities
Lentigines:	Small, flat, brown macules called "liver spots" on sun-exposed areas
Sebaceous hyperplasia:	Yellowish, flattened papular lesions with a central depression found on forehead, nose, and cheeks

Pediatric Considerations

History

Known allergies
Known exposure to communicable disease, animal or insect bites
Group settings, such as day care, school, college campus
Immunization history
Known trauma
Activity level (e.g., recently learned to walk, participation in sports)
Knowledge or suspicion of abuse

Examination

To check mobility and turgor of skin, pinch and lift a fold of skin over the abdomen.

	Normal Findings	Abnormal Findings
Infant		
	Lanugo	
	Desquamation	
	Mottling	
	Acrocyanosis	Perioral cyanosis
		Central cyanosis
	Milia	
	Erythema toxicum	
	Nevus flammeus	
	Hemangioma	Hemangioma that obstructs airway, vision
		Port wine stain
	Jaundice at approximately 2 to 14 days	Jaundice within first 48 hours and beyond second week
	Carotinemia	

	None to a full head of hair	
	Absence of axillary and pubic hair	Coarse axillary and/or pubic hair
	Mongolian spot especially in Mexican Americans	Tuft of hair or fistula over sacral area
Infant and Child		
	Café-au-lait spots: < 3; < 5 mm	Café-au-lait spots: > 3; > 5 mm
		Impetigo: honey-colored, encrusted vesicles
		Bruising in various stages of healing; unexplainable burns or wounds
Adolescent	Increasing pubic and axillary hair	
	Comedones on face back and chest	Cystic acne
		"Track" marks
	Skin alterations such as tattoos, brands	
Pregnant Female	Striae gravidarum	
	Linea nigra	
	Chloasma	
	Vascular spiders	

7

Assessment of the Head

HISTORY AND CURRENT STATUS QUESTIONS

Injury?
: Description, including any loss of consciousness and its duration, date of occurrence, precipitating or prodromal events such as faintness or pain, treatment, residual effects

Headache?
: Location, unilateral or bilateral, character and severity of pain; acute or gradual onset, pattern of occurrence (constant or chronic recurrent), worsening over time or stable in intensity, time of onset, duration, precipitating or associated factors (such as particular activities, time of day, or stressful events), effect of movement (such as change in head position, coughing, or sneezing), associated symptoms (such as nausea and vomiting, nasal congestion, or fever); relief measures tried and their effectiveness

Seizures?
: Type, sequence of seizure effects on the body, duration, postictal reaction (e.g., sleep, confusion, weakness, headache) and its duration, aura, age at onset, cause if known, frequency, any recent change in frequency, time of last seizure, exacerbating factors (e.g., stress, fatigue, specific activities, omission of

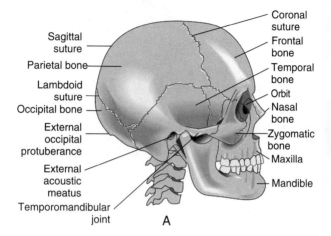

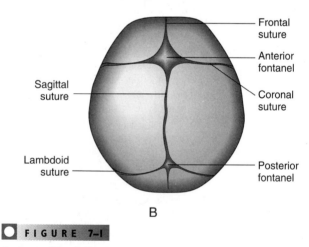

⬤ FIGURE 7–1

Anatomy of the skull.
  A, Lateral view of the adult skull.
  B, Fontanelles and bones of the infant skull.

	medication), treatment, side effects of medication, pattern of compliance with treatment regimen
Stiff neck?	Area of neck involved, any limitation of movement, date of onset, duration, constant or intermittent, precipitating or aggravating events, associated symptoms
Facial edema?	Time of onset, location, duration, associated pain, infection, medications (such as steroids), improved or worsened if currently present
Scalp problems?	Soreness, itching

PHYSICAL EXAMINATION

Equipment

Sterile pin or cotton ball

Procedures, Techniques, and Findings

Procedure	*Technique*
1. Inspect the head	Observe size, symmetry, position, and movement
2. Inspect the face	Observe size, symmetry of eyebrows, palpebral fissures, nasolabial folds, sides of the mouth, movements and facial expressions
3. Inspect scalp	Have patient remove wig or hairpiece
	Part hair in several places and observe for lesions, nits
4. Palpate the skull, noting shape, symmetry, and inconsistencies (e.g., soft spots)	

Palpate the temporal artery to check for hardness or tenderness

Use pads of index and middle fingers; locate artery below the cheek bone between the eye and the ear

5. Check function of temporo-mandibular joint

Place tip of index fingers on the sides of the face in front of the tragus of the ear and ask the patient to open the mouth; feel the fingertips slip into the joint space as the mouth opens

Note range of motion, and any swelling or tenderness

6. Test cranial nerve VII

Ask patient to smile, frown, raise eyebrows, show upper and lower teeth, keep eyes tightly closed while you try to open them (Fig. 7–2), and puff out the cheeks

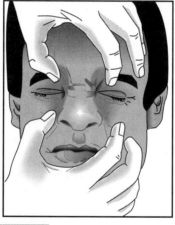

⬤ FIGURE 7–2

Testing cranial nerve VII by having patient keep the eyes tightly closed while the examiner tries to open them.

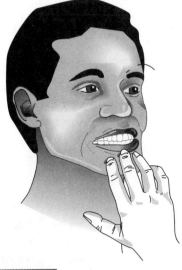

● FIGURE 7–3

Testing motor function of cranial nerve II by having patient clinch teeth as the examiner pushes down on the chin to try and separate the jaws.

	Observe for mobility and symmetry as these actions are performed
	Press puffed cheeks in and note if air escapes equally from both sides
7. Test cranial nerve V	Ask patient to clench teeth
Motor function	Push down on the chin to try and separate the jaws (Fig. 7–3)
Sensory function	Ask patient to close eyes
	Touch sterile pin or cotton ball to chin, cheeks, and forehead
	Ask patient to identify what is felt and where

	Normal Findings	Abnormal Findings
Head		
Size	Variable	Very small or very large
Symmetry	Symmetrical	Asymmetric
Position	Upright	Tilted to one side
Movement	Still except for purposeful movement	Tremors
Face		
Size and symmetry of facial features	Variable, symmetric	Excessively large or small, asymmetric, distorted lesions, masses
Facial expressions	Variable, symmetric	Distorted, absent, or asymmetric
Facial movement	Freely movable, symmetric	Distorted, absent, asymmetric
Scalp	Smooth, intact, moves freely over skull	Scaliness, lumps, redness, soft areas
Skull	Hard and smooth	Lumps, tenderness
Temporal artery	Nontender	Hard, tender
Temporomandibular joint	3 to 6 cm vertical range with mouth open 1 to 2 cm lateral motion Snapping or popping common	Pain, crepitus, restricted motion, deviation to one side upon opening the mouth
Cranial nerve VII		
Motor function	Symmetrical strength and move-	Loss of or asymmetrical movement

ment of facial
muscles

Muscle weakness
suggested by loss
of nasolabial fold,
drooping of side of
face, or drooping
of lower lid, (Fig.
7–4) no escape of
air from one or
both cheeks

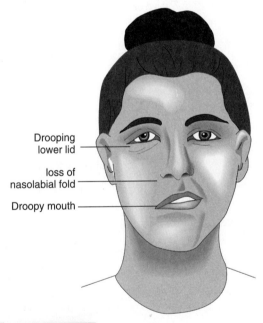

Drooping
lower lid

loss of
nasolabial fold

Droopy mouth

FIGURE 7–4

Signs of cranial nerve VII motor impairment (loss of nasolabial fold,
droopy side of face, or drooping lower lid).

Cranial nerve V

	Normal	Abnormal
Motor function	Symmetrical jaw movement	Asymmetrical jaw movement
	Equal muscle strength on left and right sides sufficient to prevent examiner from separating jaw	Unilateral or bilateral decreased strength
Sensory function	Sensations of light touch, dullness, and sharpness perceived over forehead, cheeks, and chin	Absent, decreased, or unequal sensation
	Eyelids blink when cornea touched with cotton.	Absent blink

Geriatric Considerations

Normal Findings

Head	Mild rhythmic tremors
	Prominent, tortorous temporal arteries
Face	Nose and brows prominent
	Lower face small with mouth sunken if teeth have been lost

Pediatric Considerations

History

Type of delivery?
Newborn: position assumed for sleep?
Familial large heads?

Physical Examination

EQUIPMENT

Tape measure

PROCEDURE

Measure the head circumference around the largest circumference of the cranium (i.e., over the occipital prominence, above the ears, above the eyebrows).

Palpate the size and tension of the anterior fontanelle with child upright.

Note the quality of the cry.

	Normal Findings	*Abnormal Findings*
Infant	Caput succedaneum: swelling, bruising of scalp over presenting part; swelling extends over suture lines	
	Asymmetry and flattening of occiput from newborn sleeping in one position	
	Normocephalic premature: increased occipital-frontal diameter; increased bitemporal diameter	Microcephalic Macrocephalic Hydrocephalic with "setting sun" eyes
	Fontanelle open and flat	Depressed or bulging fontanelle Dilated scalp veins
	Slight pulsation of fontanelle	
	Posterior fontanelle: approx. 2 cm (1 inch) diameter; closes 2 months	
	Anterior fontanelle: approx. 5 cm (2¼ inches) diameter; closes 12 to 18 months.	

Bulging fontanelle *only* when crying, coughing, vomiting

Tense or bulging fontanelle

Molding: sutures overlapping

Craniosynostosis: premature closing of sutures and fontanelle

Sutures palpable

Occipital prominence

Dysmorphia: abnormal facies indicative of genetic or congenital syndrome

Child

Parotid gland swelling above angle of jaw in front of ear

Erythema, tenderness of mastoid bone

CLINICAL NOTES

Always compare head circumference percentile to the percentile measurements of the previous visits.

Measure the head circumference three times and take the average.

8

Assessment of the Eye

HISTORY AND CURRENT STATUS QUESTIONS

Use of corrective lenses?	Date of last prescription change, glasses or contact lenses
	If contact lenses, type and care routines
Vision problems/changes?	Type; right, left, or both eyes; sudden or gradual onset, date first noticed; constant or intermittent; pattern of occurrence (season, time of day); relationship to near or distance vision; precipitating, exacerbating, and relieving factors; associated symptoms (these questions apply to all problems and changes below)
Double vision (diplopia)	Type (images side by side, on top of one another, or both)
Blurred vision?	Type (objects out of focus, grayness, cloudiness), area of visual field affected (entire, peripheral, central)

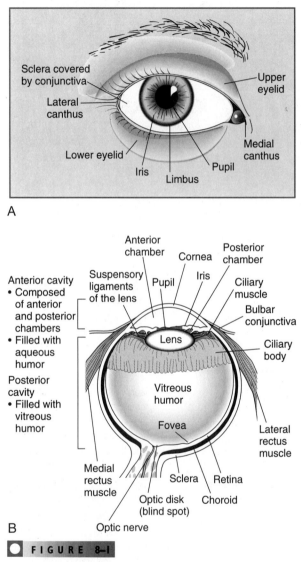

A, External eye structures. *B,* Anatomy of the eyeball.

Illustration continued on following page

● **FIGURE 8-1**

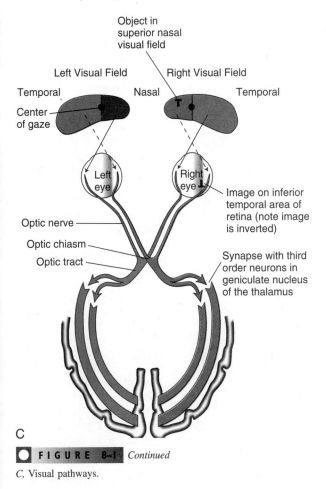

Object in
superior nasal
visual field

Left Visual Field   Right Visual Field

Temporal   Nasal   Temporal

Center
of gaze

Left
eye

Right
eye

Image on inferior
temporal area of
retina (note image
is inverted)

Optic nerve

Optic chiasm

Optic tract

Synapse with third
order neurons in
geniculate nucleus
of the thalamus

C

⬤ **FIGURE 8-1** *Continued*

C, Visual pathways.

Visual loss?   Night blindness, loss of periph-
                               eral vision, blind spots (if blind
                               spot, fixed or moving with
                               gaze)

Photophobia?	Severity
Lights/spots?	Fixed or moving, number, color, type (lightning flashes, snow flakes), halos or rings around lights
Eye pain?	Type (burning, throbbing, aching, stabbing); location (brow area, lid, surface of globe, deep in the globe); date of onset; type of onset (sudden or gradual); pattern of occurrence; precipitating, exacerbating or relieving factors; associated symptoms

External eye problems?
    Redness
    Soreness
    Burning
    Itching
    Excessive tearing
    Excessive dryness
    Discharge
	Type, location, date of onset, type of onset (sudden or gradual), constant or intermittent, associated symptoms, treatment utilized, response to treatment

Life-style factors	Type of work normally done; type of lighting used; exposure to industrial hazards, fumes, flying objects; participation in sports; use of protective goggles
Previous eye disorders, surgery, or trauma	Type, date of occurrence, treatment, residual effects
Last eye/glaucoma examination	Date, purpose, findings
History of systemic disorders affecting the eye	Diabetes, hypertension, HIV, thyroid disorder, allergies

PHYSICAL EXAMINATION

Equipment

Snellen chart, near-vision chart, or newsprint
Cover card
Pen light
Ophthalmoscope (Fig. 8–2)

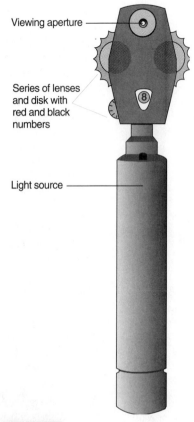

Viewing aperture

Series of lenses
and disk with
red and black
numbers

Light source

● FIGURE 8–2

Opthalmoscope.

Procedures, Techniques, and Findings

Procedure

Technique

1. Test visual acuity
   Distance vision

Position the patient 20 feet in front of a Snellen chart

Direct him or her to cover the left eye and read the smallest line of print possible

Record acuity as 20 (distance from chart) over the number found alongside the smallest line of print the patient can read with at least half the letters correct; add to this ratio a minus sign and the number of letters in the line missed by the patient (e.g., 20/30-2, patient can read at 20 feet with errors on two letters what a person with normal vision can read at 30)

Repeat for the right eye

If corrective lenses are worn, test with and then without them. Record CC next to result with corrective lenses, SC next to result without them

If patient cannot see letters, test for finger-counting ability, hand motion, and light perception as described under clinical notes

   Near vision (done for those over 40 or with complaints of reading difficulty)

Ask the patient to read the smallest letters possible (with reading glasses if worn) from a Joeger chart placed 14 inches in front of the face

Record results as J1 through
J12 (the largest letters)
indicated on the chart

Alternatively, have the patient
hold and read from material
such as a piece of newsprint at
a comfortable distance from
the face; document in the
record the type of reading material and the measured distance held from the face

2. Examine outer eye structure
   to observe position of eye
   lids in relationship to the
   globe

Note any visible sclera above
the iris

3. Observe the globe

Note alignment and position
relative to the bony orbit

Inspect the lids

Note closure, size, and presence of lesions or tics

Inspect the lashes

Note distribution, thickness, condition, and direction of lashes

*Inspect the sclera and
conjunctiva*

Separate the lids between the
index finger and the thumb
(Fig. 8–3A)

Ask the patient to look up,
down, and to each side

Note color, vascular pattern,
and presence of lesions

Inspect the palpebral conjunctiva of lower lids by asking
the patient to look up while
you evert the lid with your
thumb (Fig.8–3B)

*Check the clarity of the
cornea*

Shine a light from the side
onto each eye and observe
smoothness as well as for
cloudiness and opacities

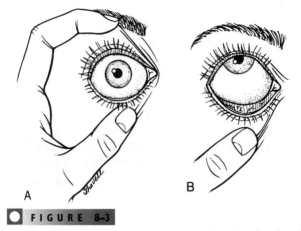

FIGURE 8–3

A, Inspection of the sclera. *B*, Inspection of the palpebral conjunctiva of the lower lid.

Inspect each iris	Compare the appearance of both irises in terms of shape, color, clarity, and markings
Inspect the pupil	Note dilatation or constriction, shape, and symmetry between the right and the left
Test the pupillary response to light	Direct the patient to look ahead off into the distance; shine a bright light on each pupil in turn, bringing it from the side to directly in front of the pupil
	Observe for constriction of the pupil into which the light is shown (direct response) and for the simultaneous constriction of the other pupil (consensual response); note size of pupils prior to exposure to light, then after constriction

(e.g., 4mm to 2mm); compare the amount and speed (e.g., brisk or sluggish) of constriction and subsequent dilatation in the two eyes

Test for accommodation

Hold your finger, a pen, or other similar object 10 to 15 cm (4 to 6 inches) from the patient's nose

Direct the patient to look off into the distance behind you and then look quickly at the finger

Observe for convergence (medial movement of both eyes) and pupillary constriction (Fig. 8–4).

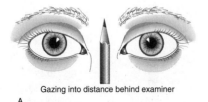

Gazing into distance behind examiner

A.

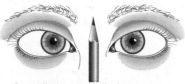

Gaze shifted to pen resulting in convergence and pupillary constriction

B.

● FIGURE 8–4

Test for accommodation.

A, Gazing into distance behind the examiner.

B, Gaze shifted to pen, resulting in convergence and pupillary construction.

3. Test extraocular muscle
   function

   Check for parallel gaze   Direct the patient to look
   (corneal light reflex)   straight ahead

                                      Shine a light into the patient's
                                      eyes from a distance of 31
                                      cm (12 inches); note the loca-
                                      tion of the light reflection on
                                      the corneas

   Assess for coordinated   Direct the patient to hold the
   movement of the two   head still and follow your
   eyes   finger with his or her eyes as it
                                      moves

                                      Hold your finger about 31 cm
                                      (12 inches) in front of the
                                      patient and move it through
                                      the cardinal fields of gaze

                                      Move your finger from the
                                      center out to one of the eight
                                      positions shown in Figure 8–5,
                                      hold it momentarily, and bring
                                      it back to the center

                                      Progress to each of the
                                      remaining positions, moving in
                                      a clockwise fashion

                                      Observe for parallel eye
                                      movement

                                      Observe relationship of upper
                                      eye lid to the iris as the gaze
                                      moves up to down

   Check for convergence   Ask the patient to watch your
                                      finger as it is moved from
                                      directly in front of the eye in
                                      toward the bridge of the nose

4. Perform the confrontation   Position yourself so you have
   test for a gross check of vi-   the same visual field as the
   sual fields   patient: put your face in front

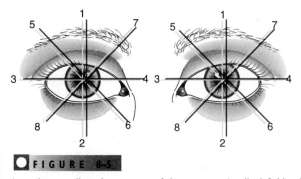

FIGURE 8-5

Assessing coordinated movement of the two eyes (cardinal fields of gaze).

of and on a level with the patient's face; ask the patient to cover his or her right eye and with his or her left eye look into your right eye; and close or cover your left eye

Bring a raised finger, pen, or other similar object held at arm's length midway between you and the patient, from the right periphery into the visual field in several directions

Direct the patient to say "Now" when the object comes into sight

Compare the time the patient sees it with when you see it

Repeat the above bringing the object into the field of vision from the left periphery

Repeat entire procedure for the opposite eye

5. Examine the ocular fundus (retina, optic disk, macula, and retinal vessels)

Perform the examination in a darkened room using an opthalmoscope

Use your right eye to examine the patient's right eye; use your left eye to examine the patient's left eye

Position yourself about 15 inches away from the patient and slightly to the side of his or her line of vision

Select a large round aperture with white light and place the opthalmoscope with lens set at zero diopters firmly under the medial aspect of your orbit and shine the light beam on the pupil of the eye to be examined

Tell the patient to keep looking or staring at a spot across the room

Note the red reflex (orange-red glow in the pupil) and note any areas of opacity interrupting it

Maintain focus on the red reflex while you move your head and the ophthalmoscope forward as a unit until it almost touches the patient's eye lashes

Rotate the lens disk to focus on the optic disk (yellow-orange to creamy-pink round or oval area upon which the blood vessels of the retina converge) of the retina

Locate the optic disk (Fig. 8–6), which is found to the nasal side of the retina, by following a blood vessel in the direction in which it enlarges and has branches joining it

Note size, shape, clarity, and color of the disk margins

Inspect the physiologic cup, including its central depression, and note the cup–disk ratio. Also note the emerging retinal arterioles and veins (arterioles are light red with a bright reflection; veins are dark red, without reflection, and one-fourth to one-third larger than arterioles)

Observe the branching pattern, fullness, contour, and integrity of the vessels

Proceed to the peripheral retina

Locate the macula

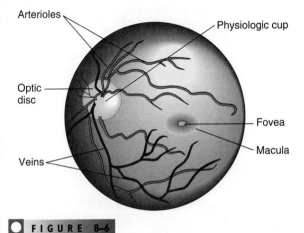

Arterioles

Physiologic cup

Optic disc

Fovea

Macula

Veins

⬤ FIGURE 8-6

Normal ocular fundus, left eye.

	Normal Findings	**Abnormal Findings**
Visual acuity		
Distance vision	20/20 in each eye	Less than 20/20 (i.e., 20/30 or higher with correction, 20/200 with correction in either eye is legal blindness)
Near vision	J1 or 14/14 in each eye read without moving the card and without hesitancy	J2 or higher or less than 14/14
Outer eye structures		
Eye lids	No sclera visible between upper lid and iris Upper and lower lids completely approximated when closed Skin intact and free of erythema, edema, discharge, and lesions	Visible sclera above the iris, incomplete closure, ptosis or drooping of the upper lid, erythema, edema, discharge, or lesions
Eye lashes	Evenly distributed with an outward curve	Uneven distribution crusting, brushing the globe
Globe	Evenly aligned and neither sunken nor protruding	Uneven alignment, sunken or protruberant

Conjunctiva and sclera	Sclera smooth, white, glossy, and moist	Generalized yellow or red discoloration, pallor near outer canthus, cyanosis of lower lid, bulging, inflammation, nodules, discharge
	Small brown macules, grey-blue tinge, and/or yellow areas under lids common in blacks	
	Clear, pale glistening pink conjunctiva, numerous small visible blood vessels common	
Pupil	Round, regular, 3 to 5 mm, equal in both eyes	Excessively dilated or constricted, irregular, unequal (Table 8–1)
	Difference in size seen occasionally as a normal variation	
Pupillary response to light	Symmetrical constriction followed by symmetrical dilation in terms of amount and speed	
	Response recorded in millimeters (e.g., R3/1 = 3/1L)	Absence of constriction, asymmetrical response
	nominator = resting size = 3 mm	
	denominator = size in response to light = 1 mm	
Accommodation	Convergence of both eyes	Absence of convergence, asymmetrical response

TABLE 8–1
Variations and Abnormalities of the Pupil

Variation/ Abnormality	Description	Etiology
Anisocoria	Pupils are unequal in size	Normal in small percentage of the population Central nervous system disease
Monocular	Absence of pupillary response to light directed to the blind eye with bilateral pupillary constriction in response to light shown in the normal eye	Blindness in one eye with an intact oculomotor nerve
Miosis	Constricted, fixed pupils	Iritis, damage to the pons, use of narcotics, use of pilocarpine
Mydriasis	Dilated, fixed pupils	Acute glaucoma, trauma, CNS disease, sympathetic nervous system stimulation, use of sympathomimetic drugs or pupillary dilating drops, deep anesthesia, or cardiac arrest

Table continued on following page

TABLE 8-1
Variations and Abnormalities of the Pupil *Continued*

Variation/ Abnormality	Description	Etiology
Argyll-Robertson pupil	No constriction in response to light or accommodation	Chronic alcoholism, third-stage syphilis, meningitis, intracranial tumor
Tonic pupil	Large, regular pupil with a sluggish reaction to light and accommodation	Normal variation, which is usually unilateral
Cranial nerve III impaired *Pupil*	Deviation of one eye downward and to the side, accompanied by a dilated pupil nonreactive to light or accommodation and by ptosis of the lid	Damage to the oculomotor nerve
Horner syndrome	Small, regular pupil reactive to light and accommodation accompanied by ipsilateral ptosis and anhidrosis	Sympathetic nerve damage, unilateral

Extraocular muscles

Parallel gaze	Reflections of light on the cornea are on or just medial to the pupil in both eyes	Reflections of light are in different locations in each eye
Coordinated movement of	Eye movement when tracking objects is parallel	Nonparallel eye movement, failure to follow in a certain direction; nystagmus at other than the end point of gaze
	Upper lid overlaps iris at all times as the gaze moves from up to down	
	Occasional nystagmus at end point of gaze	Lid lag—appearance of a white rim of sclera between the lid and the iris
Convergence	Sustained to within 5 to 8 cm	
Confrontation visual field test	Patient's visual field same as examiner's, provided examiner's is normal. Noted as "visual fields full to confrontation"	Patient's visual field less than examiner's. Noted as "Unable to detect ___ cm object on upper, outer quadrant of visual field OD" (or OS)

Ocular fundus

Red reflex	Uninterrupted red glow filling the pupil	Dark shadows or black dots interrupting the red glow
Optic disk	Yellow-orange to	Dark color (seen

	creamy pink, round or oval, distinct sharp margins except for nasal edge, which is sometimes blurred	with eye strain and astigmatism); pale or white color (seen with glaucoma or optic atrophy)
Retinal vessels	Paired artery and vein passing to each quadrant, ratio of arterial diameter 2:3 or 4:5, regular decrease in diameter of veins and arteries as they progress to the periphery, mild vessel twisting, artery and vein crossings within 2 disk diameters (DD) of disk, no interruption of blood flow, no indenting or displacing of vessels	Absence of major vessels, arteries constricted, veins dilated, neovascularization, extreme vessel tortuosity or asymmetrical tortuosity in the two eyes, artery and vein crossings more than 2 DD from disk, vessels engorged peripheral to the crossing
Retina	Light red to dark brown-red with shade corresponding to skin color, free of lesions	Areas of hemorrhage, exudate, altered color, microaneurysms
Macula	One disk diameter (1 DD) in size Even, homogenous color, may be slightly darker than rest of fundus	Hemorrhage, exudate, clumps of pigment

■ **T A B L E   8–2**
**Common Variations and Abnormalities
of the Eye**

Variation/ Abnormality	Description and Significance	Illustration
Retracted upper lid	Rim of white sclera is visible above the iris	
Ptosis	Drooping of the upper eyelid; may be due to age-related or pathological muscle weakness or nerve impairment	
Ectropion	Outward sagging of the lower lid, which can lead to skin excoriation and corneal ulceration; may be congenital, age-related or due to cranial nerve VII palsy	
Entropion	Turning inward of the eyelid due to aging, chronic inflammation, or scarring; may result in lashes touching globe, causing pain (age effect seen in lower lid only)	
Herniated fat	Bulging of lower lids and/or inner third of upper due to fat displacing weakened lid fascia forward; occurs most often in the elderly	
Pinguecula	Benign creamy-yellow triangular nodule on the conjunctiva on either side of the iris	

Table continued on following page

TABLE 8–2
Common Variations and Abnormalities
of the Eye *Continued*

Variation/ Abnormality	Description and Significance	Illustration
Chalazion	Chronic inflammation of the meibomian gland that appears as a painless nodule usually involving the conjunctival side of the lid	
Hordeolum (sty)	Painful, red, pimple-like area of infection on the lid/lash margin	
Xanthelasma	Clearly demarcated raised, yellow plaques in the skin of the nasal portion of the eyelid; associated in some cases with lipid disorder	
Pterygium	Triangular thickening of the bulbar conjunctiva, usually on the nasal side, which may grow across the iris	
Arcus senilis (corneal arcus)	Opaque white or gray ring around the iris; occurs with normal aging though also is seen in younger persons	
Conjunctivitis	Inflammation or infection of the conjunctiva characterized by increased prominence of blood vessels, redness that is greatest at the periphery, discomfort, and discharge	

Table continued on following page

TABLE 8–2
Common Variations and Abnormalities of the Eye *Continued*

Variation/ Abnormality	Description and Significance	Illustration
Subconjunctival hemorrhage	Sharply delineated deep-red area that slowly turns to yellow and disappears; may be due to trauma, action causing a sudden venous pressure increase, or a bleeding disorder	
Corneal scar	Superficial gray-white opaque area in the cornea due to previous trauma/inflammation	
Cataract	Opacity of the lens that appears gray when seen through the pupil with a flashlight or black against the red reflex when seen through an ophthalmoscope	

TABLE 8–3
Common Variations and Abnormalities of the Optic Disc

Variation/ Abnormality	Description and Significance	Illustration
Optic atrophy	Loss of tiny vessels due to death of optic nerve fibers	

Table continued on following page

T A B L E   8–3
Common Variations and Abnormalities of the Optic Disc *Continued*

Variation/ Abnormality	Description and Significance	Illustration
Papilledema	Engorment and elevation of the disc with blurred disc margins due to venous stasis secondary to increased intracranial pressure	
Neovascularization	Growth of new blood vessels that are narrow, tortuous, and more numerous than surrounding vessels; associated with diabetic retinopathy	
Cotton wool patches (soft exudates)	Grayish white oval lesions with irregular margins associated with hypertension	
Hard exudates	Creamy-yellow well-demarcated lesions that may be discrete, small and round, or large and irregular because of coalescence; associated with diabetes and hypertension	

Clinical Notes

Use an eye chart with rows of numbers or E's pointing in varying directions for patients unable to identify letters. Check the patient's ability to count the number of fingers held up by the examiner if no lines on a Snellen chart can be read. When 50% or more finger presentations are

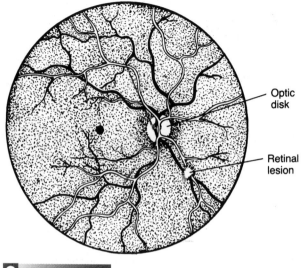

Optic
disk

Retinal
lesion

FIGURE 8-7

Position of lesion on ocular fundus.

identified correctly document the patient's performance
on this counting fingers test as "Counts fingers at
_____ feet."

Test ability to perceive hand motion in patients unable to
count fingers. Do this by having the patient cover each
eye in turn and waving your hand either up or down
or right to left. When the patient correctly identifies the
direction of the hand wave 50% of the time, document
the results as "Hand motion at _____ feet."

Test light perception if the patient is unable to detect hand
motion. Darken the room and direct the patient to cover
one eye. Shine a bright light into the uncovered eye at
random intervals, turning it off between them. Ask the
patient to report when light is seen. Document the patient
as having light-perception acuity if 50% of the light
presentations are identified. Repeat for the other eye.

If a near vision chart cannot be used, estimate near vision by using any printed material.

Record normal pupillary findings as PERRLA (pupils equal, round, reactive to light, and accommodation).

Document findings in the ocular fundus by noting clock position and relation to the optic disk in terms of size and distance. For example "_____ noted at 1 o'clock, 1½ DD from the disk" (Fig. 8–7).

Geriatric Considerations

Additional History Questions

Family history of cataracts?

Date of last glaucoma test?

Problems with night vision, glare, distinguishing colors?

Loss of peripheral or central vision?

Burning or dryness of eyes?

Problems with management of eye drops (if applicable)?

	Normal Findings
Visual acuity	20/20 to 20/70 distance vision some blurriness on near vision (presbyopia)
External eye structures	Thin outer aspect of eyebrows due to a decrease in hair follicles
	Wrinkled, baggy lids and wrinkling of skin around eyes due to atrophy
	Bulging of lower lids and/or inner third of upper lids due to pressure of fat on atrophied fascia
	Partial ptosis of upper lid due to muscle atrophy
	Xanthalasma (benign, soft, yellow plaques on lids at inner canthus)
	Sunken because of loss of supporting fat
	Dry because of decreased tear production

Entropion: turning inward of lower lid

or

Ectropion: drooping of the lid away from the globe due to atrophy of elastic and fibrous tissue

Globe

Arcus senilis (white to gray circle around the outer edge of the cornea due to the deposition of lipid and without clinical significance)

Clouding, dullness of the cornea

Decreased pupil size and occasional slight irregularity

Slowed pupillary light reflex

Fundus

Less shiny

Pale, narrow, straight arterioles

Increased number of A–V crossing defects

Drusen (hyaline deposits that appear as small, scattered, round, yellow spots on the retina); may occur with normal aging but may also indicate early macular degeneration

Vitreous floaters

Pediatric Considerations

History

Maternal rubella?
Squinting, rubbing eyes?
Holding books near to face, sitting close to TV?

Physical Examination

EQUIPMENT.

Snellen pre-school picture chart

PROCEDURE.

Check red reflex in all newborns.

Note spacing and symmetry of eyes.

"Cover test" by age 1 year: cover one eye, uncover suddenly and observe for an abnormal shift from a lateral or medial to a central gaze.

Visual acuity test by 3 years of age.

Normal Findings	Common Variations	Abnormal Findings
Newborn, Infant, and Child		
		Wide-set eyes
		Palpebral slant in non-Asian
		Epicanthal folds
Red-orange reflex		Abnormal red reflex; opacity
Intermittent convergent strabismus < 6 months		Divergent strabismus
Corneal reflex		Asymmetry of red reflex on pupil
Direct consensual pupillary constriction in response to bright light		
Visual acuity:		
4 weeks: fixation on object		
6 weeks: follows < 180 degrees		
4 months: follows > 180 degrees; convergence		

1 year: 20/200;
focuses; hand-
eye coordination

3 years: 20/40

5 years: 20/30

6 to 7 years:
20/20   Ptosis

Chemical conjunc-
tivitis (from instil-
lation of medica-
tion in delivery
room)

Small subconjunc-
tival and scleral
hemorrhage

Lacrimal meatus
obstructed, with
tearing and mu-
cous collecting in
the eye

Pseudostrabismus
secondary to wide
bridge of nose

Clinical Notes

Refer to an ophthalmologist before visual acuity test at 3
years if child has an opacity of lens, does not follow gaze,
demonstrates divergent strabismus, fails "cover test," or
presents with dilated, tortuous, retinal vessels.

9

Assessment of the Ear

HISTORY AND CURRENT STATUS QUESTIONS

Hearing loss?

Unilateral or bilateral; date first noticed; sudden or gradual onset (if gradual over what time span); general or selective loss (e.g., high sounds, conversational tones when background noise is present); severity; precipitating or associated factors; effects on daily activities, job responsibilities, and social interactions; use of hearing aid, including type and effectiveness

Ear pain or discomfort?

Unilateral or bilateral, date and type of onset, constant or intermittent, type (throbbing, feeling of fullness, dull ache, sharp, stabbing), location (outer ear or deep in the head), changes in the type of pain since onset, precipitating or worsening factors (changing the position of the head, pulling or pushing on the ear, chewing, yawning, or exposure to heat or cold) type and effectiveness of treatment measures utilized, associated symptoms

Discharge?

Unilateral or bilateral, date and type of onset (sudden or gradual), color, odor, consistency, amount, constant or intermittent, precipitating

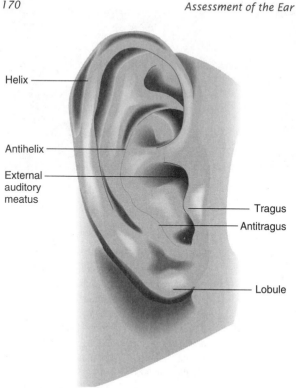

FIGURE 9-1

Anatomy of the Ear

	factors, associated symptoms (skin irritation, canal itching, fever, pain)
Tinnitus?	Unilateral or bilateral, date of onset, quality (high- or low-pitched, roaring, humming, or hissing), severity, constant or intermittent, precipitating factors, long-term use of aspirin or other salicylates (how much, how often, for how long)

Vertigo?	Time and type of onset, severity, constant or intermittent, associated symptoms (nausea, vomiting, ataxia), precipitating factors, type and effectiveness of relief measures used
	Be certain to differentiate vertigo, in which the room is perceived as moving around, from dizziness, in which the patient feels the movement
Last hearing examination?	Date, type, reason for, by whom
Use of a hearing aid or other assistive devices?	Type of device used, consistency of use, perceived effectiveness, care of device, difficulties with the device
Prior ear problems?	Type (surgery, trauma, infections, etc.) date(s), treatment, residual effects
Exposure to ototoxic factors?	Use of medications such as aspirin, gentomicin and other aminoglycosides, quinine, ethycrinic acid, furosemide and vancomycin
	Long-term exposure to loud noise (e.g., from traffic, machinery, gunshots, radios, concerts)
Related health problems?	Allergies; colds; sinus, eye, mouth, teeth, jaw, or throat problems; recent head trauma
Self-care routines related to the ear?	Hygienic practices, use of protective head phones or ear plugs

PHYSICAL EXAMINATION

Equipment

Otoscope (Fig. 9–2) with fresh batteries so white, not yellow light is produced

Tuning fork (512 or 1024 Hz)

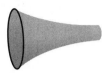

Ear specula

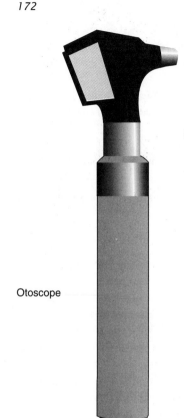

Otoscope

FIGURE 9–2

Otoscope

Procedures, Techniques, and Findings

Procedure	*Technique*
1. Inspect the external ear	Note placement, size, shape, symmetry and skin color
	Observe for drainage, swelling, lumps and skin lesions

2. Palpate the external ear

Feel for nodules or other irregularities

Move the pinna up and down,
push on the tragus, and press
behind the ear

3. Inspect the external auditory
   meatus

Note the size of the opening,
and look for any redness,
swelling, discharge, or foreign
body

4. Examine the external auditory canal and ear drum
   with an otoscope

Have patient assume a sitting
position

Use largest speculum that fits
comfortably in the auditory
canal

Position self to the side and
slightly to the back of the ear
to be examined

Ask the patient to tip his or her
head toward the shoulder opposite the ear being examined

Using the nondominant hand
grasp the pinna at the top and
pull it up, back and slightly
away from the head to
straighten the adult ear canal;
maintain this position until the
otoscope is removed

Hold the otoscope in the dominant hand in an upside-down
position; brace your hand
against the patient's head so
that if the patient's head
moves, your hand and the otoscope also move (Fig. 9–3)

Insert the speculum into the
canal (½ inch) slowly, angling

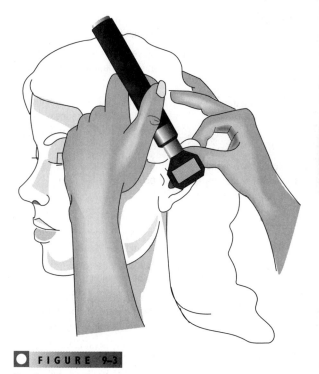

● FIGURE 9–3

Routine when using otoscope

it slightly downward and
forward

Avoid touching the medial wall
of the canal, as it is sensitive
to pain

Observe the auditory canal for
ear wax, swelling, redness,
discharge, foreign bodies, lesions

Inspect the ear drum; note color, contour, intactness

(If the ear drum is not seen, reposition the patient's head; exert more pull on the pinna; and angle the otoscope more forward)

Observe the position of the handle of the malleus, the umbo, the short process, and the cone of light. Rotate the otoscope as needed to visualize all areas of the ear drum (Fig. 9–4)

Clean off any discharge or change the speculum and repeat for the other ear

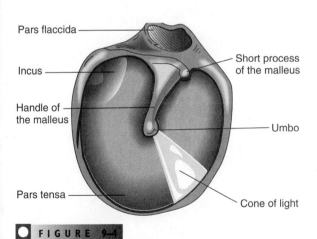

Pars flaccida

Incus

Handle of the malleus

Short process of the malleus

Umbo

Pars tensa

Cone of light

FIGURE 9–4

Ear drum

5. Test hearing acuity (cranial nerve VIII)

Position self 1 to 2 feet from patient

Gross acuity

Voice test: Occlude one ear by placing your index finger in the external meatus and moving it back and forth gently but rapidly

Position self 1 to 2 feet from the patient

Exhale completely and with your mouth covered or the patient's eyes closed to prevent lip reading, whisper words of two equally accented syllables (baseball, arm chair) toward the ear being tested

Repeat for other ear

Lateralization of sound

Weber test: Set a tuning fork of 512 or 1024 Hz lightly vibrating by tapping the tines against your other hand (Fig. 9–5A)

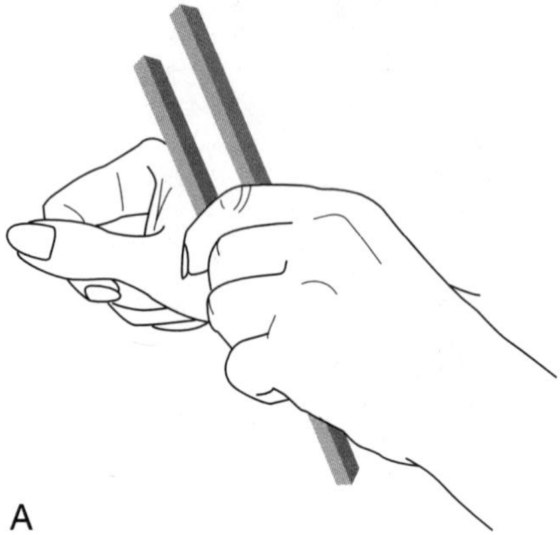

A

● FIGURE 9–5

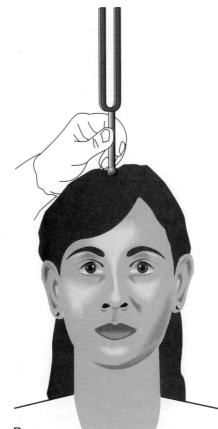

B

⬤ FIGURE 9-5 *Continued*

A and *B* Weber test

Place the base of the vibrating tuning fork on top of the patient's head or in the middle of the forehead (Fig. 9–5*B*).

Ask the patient where the tone is heard: right ear, left ear, or both; if both, ask if loudness is equal on both sides

Comparison of air and bone conduction

Rinne test: Place the base of a lightly vibrating tuning fork on the mastoid process (Fig. 9–6*A*)

Ask patient to say when the tone is no longer heard

When the patient no longer hears the tone quickly, move the fork so the tines are in front of the auditory meatus (Fig. 9-6*B*)

Ask patient if a tone is heard and direct him or her to indicate when it ends

Repeat with other ear

A

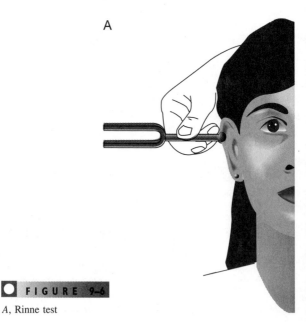

FIGURE 9–6

A, Rinne test

B

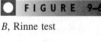

FIGURE 9–6 *Continued*

B, Rinne test

	Normal Findings	**Abnormal Findings**
External Ear		
Placement	Top of pinna level with outer corner of the eye; ear angled <10 degrees toward occiput	Top of pinna below level of outer corner of the eye Unequal alignment
Size	Variable but equal (4 to 10 cm)	Excessively large or undeveloped Unequal
General appearance	Skin intact, similar in color to face, smooth, uniform	Lesions, erythema, cyanosis, edema, masses, drainage

Findings on palpation	Pinna, tragus, and mastoid nontender on manipulation; well-defined bony edges on the mastoid process	Tenderness or pain on manipulation of pinna, tragus, or mastoid
External auditory meatus	Patent	Obstructed
Auditory canal	Walls pink and uniform Cilia and cerumen (wet cerumen, which is honey-colored to dark brown, or black and moist in most whites and blacks, or dry cerumen, which is gray and flaky in most Asians and Native Americans).	Marked pain on insertion of the speculum, discharge, foul odor, edema, erythema, flaking, lesions, excessive build-up of cerumen, foreign body, complete obstruction (Table 9–1)
Tympanic membrane	Intact, pearly gray, shiny, translucent, conical, landmarks (cone of light at 5 o'clock in right ear and 7 o'clock in left, umbo, handle of malleus, and the short process) clearly visible	Perforated or scarred, dull, blue or red, yellow-amber, retraction accentuated landmarks, bulging drum with partially occluded landmarks (Table 9–2)
	Flutters when patient holds nose and swallows	No movement of tympanic membrane when patient holds the nose and swallows

TABLE 9-1
Variations and Abnormalities of the External Ear

Location	Variation/Abnormality	Description and Significance
Helix	Tophi	Deposits of uric acid crystals that appear as hard, white to yellow, painless nodules Associated with gout, a painful metabolic bone disorder
	Darwin's tubercle	Small painless elevation typically toward top of helix Benign, congenital variation
	Chondrodermatitis	Small painful, indurated nodule of unknown etiology Most common in men
Ear canal	Otitis externa	Tender, inflamed canal Narrowed by swelling
	Furuncle	Infected hair follicle, which appears as a red, elevated, exquisitely tender nodule and is frequently accompanied by regional lymphadenopathy
	Polyp	Benign tumor that is red and bleeds readily
	Osteoma	Benign nontender, rock-hard, round nodule covered with apparently normal skin occurring in the inner third of the canal and obscuring the ear drum
	Exostosis	Multiple hard, round nodules of bone covered with epithelium that occur near the tympanic membrane in both ears

TABLE 9–2
Abnormal Otoscopy Findings

Appearance of Eardrum	Indicates
Yellow-amber color	Serum or pus
Prominent landmarks	Retraction of drum
Air/fluid level or air bubbles	Serous fluid
Absent or distorted light reflex	Bulging of eardrum
Bright red color	Infection in middle ear
Blue or dark red color	Blood behind drum
Dark oval areas	Perforation
White dense areas	Scarring
Diminished or absent landmarks	Thickened drum
Black or white dots on drum or canal	Colony growth

Voice test (gross hearing acuity)	Able to repeat words whispered at a distance of 1 to 2 feet	Unable to hear whispered words
Weber test (lateralization of sound)	Vibratory tone heard equally in both ears	Tone lateralized to affected ear in conductive hearing loss and to unaffected ear in sensorineural hearing loss
Rinne test (comparison of air to bone conduction)	Air conduction twice as long as bone conduction	Air conduction equal to or shorter than bone conduction in conductive hearing loss
		Air conduction longer (but not twice as long) as bone conduction in sensorineural hearing loss

Clinical Notes

Observe for signs of hearing loss during all interactions with the patient. These include a flat, monotonous tone or very loud voice, posturing of the head to direct sound to the preferred ear, the appearance of intense concentration and straining to hear, focus on the face and lips rather than the eyes of the speaker, and frequently misunderstand directions and questions or requests to repeat them.

Check the external auditory canal of all patients who wear hearing aids for irritation from badly fitting earmolds.

Never insert a speculum if a foreign object is seen in the external canal.

Geriatric Considerations

History

Wear or have worn a hearing aid? Proper fit?
History of perforated tympanic membrane?
History of cerumen impaction?

	Normal Findings
Ear lobes	Pendulous with linear wrinkling due to loss of elasticity
	Hair growth on helix, antihelix, and tragus of pinna
External meatus	Coarse, stiff hairs at entrance
Cerumen	Drier than usual because of apocrine gland atrophy
Tympanic membrane	Whiter, duller, and thicker than in younger adult
Hearing	Presbycusis: sensory neural hearing loss characterized by initial inability to hear high-pitched tones, difficulty distinguishing consonant sounds as opposed to vowel sounds
Auditory reaction time	Increased (i.e., takes longer "to hear" and to respond)

Pediatric Considerations

History

Known congenital hearing loss in other family members?
History of chronic and/or recurrent otitis?
Method of cleaning the child's ears?
History of child placing foreign objects in the ear?
Language development age appropriate?
Child's response to normal conversational tones?
Caretaker's intuitive feeling about the child's hearing?

Physical Examination

EQUIPMENT.

Otoscope with gradient-size speculum
Pneumatic tube (an otoscope attachment that allows air to
  be introduced into and removed from the ear canal for
  the purpose of altering pressure on the tympanic
  membrane and thus assessing its vibrability)

PROCEDURE.

To examine the internal ear of an infant pull the pinna
  downward since the ear canal is directed downward. To
  examine the internal ear of a child pull the pinna up, out,
  and back since the canal is directed upward and backward.
Securely restrain children, either on the caretaker's lap or
  an examining table, so as to prevent head movement
  during examination of the internal ear.

	Normal Findings	*Abnormal Findings*
Infant	Normal placement and alignment: pinna of both ears joins head at or above an imaginary line drawn across the inner and outer canthus of each eye	Low-set ears Deviation in alignment
	Preauricular skin tag	Preauricular dimple Unilateral or bilateral

	malformation (may indicate other defects)
Tympanic membrane mobile (moves inward when air is introduced into the canal and outward when ear air is removed via a pneumatic tube)	Tympanic membrane immobile
Sound produces:	Absence of normal response to sound
Birth: Acoustic blink reflex	
2 weeks: Moro (startle) reflex	
10 weeks: Cessation of movement	
3 to 4 months: Turning toward sound	

Child and Adolescent

Selective deafness	External otitis, ("swimmer's ear"): pain upon movement of pinna

Clinical Notes

Although multiple variables affect speech development, the following milestones are assessed:

2 months: Cooing
4 months: Babbling, squealing
9 months: Polysyllabic vocalizing
1 year: Single words
2 years: Multiple-word vocabulary; combining two words

10

Assessment of the Nose and Sinuses

HISTORY AND CURRENT STATUS QUESTIONS

Rhinorrhea? Nasal stuffiness? Sneezing?	Unilateral or bilateral, pattern of occurrence: days' duration; during cold and flu season or seasonal; intermittent or continuous; associated contacts or environments; character and amount of drainage; remedies used and their effectiveness; use of drugs that cause stuffiness such as oral contraceptives, reserpine, guanethidine and alcohol; associated symptoms such as facial pain, headache, and fever
Epistaxis?	Severity, duration, associated symptoms, recurrent, other bleeding or easy bruising, any medications taken such as aspirin or warfarin
Changes in appetite or sense of smell?	Time of onset, type of change, worsened or improved with time
Allergies?	Type, treatment and its effectiveness
URIs?	Type, frequency, duration, treatment
Use of nasal sprays?	Type, how often, for what reason

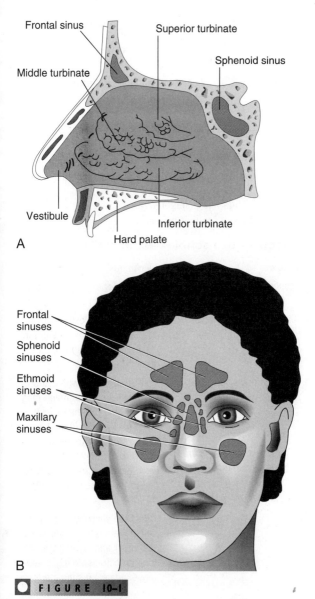

FIGURE 10–1

A. Anatomy of the Nasal Cavity
B. Facial Sinuses (frontal view)

| Surgery or trauma? | Type, date of occurrence, residual effects |
| Sinus pain? | Location, severity, duration, treatment utilized, effectiveness of treatment |

PHYSICAL EXAMINATION

Equipment

Otoscope with a short, wide nasal tip and a magnifying lens or

Nasal speculum and penlight

Small vials with familiar odors

Procedures, Techniques, and Findings

Procedure	*Technique*
1. Inspect the external aspect of the nose	Observe for asymmetry, deformity, lesions or inflammation
2. Check patency of nares	Ask patient to close mouth then occlude each naris in turn Feel for exhaled air from the nonoccluded naris
3. Inspect the inside of the nose *Mucosa* *Nasal septum* *Inferior and middle turbinates and middle meatus between them*	Use an otoscope with a short, wide nasal speculum and magnifying lens. Tilt the patient's head back and hold the handle of the otoscope to the side. Insert the speculum 1 cm into each naris in turn, taking care not to touch the septum (Fig. 10-2) Direct the speculum back and somewhat up to visualize both the upper and lower nose; look for color, swelling, bleeding, exudate, crusting, perforation or deviation of the septum, polyps on the turbinates, and foreign bodies

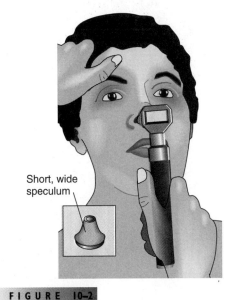

● FIGURE 10–2

Examine naris

4. Palpate the sinuses for tenderness

Frontal sinus

Using pads of thumbs, press up from under the medial aspect of the brow ridges (Fig. 10–3*A*).

Maxillary sinus

Place pads of thumbs under the zygomatic arch then press up and in (Fig. 10–3*B*).

5. Test cranial nerve I

Ask patient to close eyes; occlude one naris and hold a substance with a familiar odor beneath the other; ask the patient if anything is smelled and, if so, what it is

Repeat for other side

Short, wide speculum

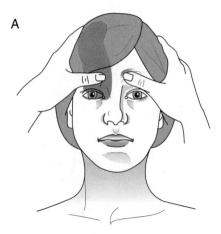

FIGURE 10-3

A and *B* Palpating sinuses

	Normal Findings	**Abnormal Findings**
External nose	Symmetrical	Asymmetrical, watery, purulent, mucous or bloody discharge; crusting,

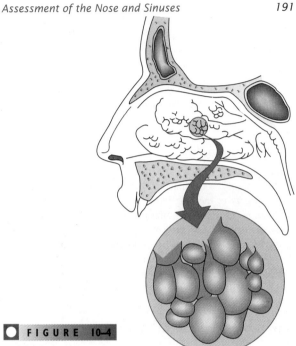

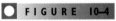

FIGURE 10–4

Nasal polyps

		nasal flaring, bullous, visible vasculature, erythema
Patency of nares	Air felt when exhaled	Noise or absence of air upon exhalation
Nasal mucosa	Intact, smooth, moist pink (deeper color than oral mucosa)	Pallor, bright red or gray color, swelling, bogginess, exudate, bleeding fissures, ulcers, polyps (Fig. 10–4), tenderness

Nasal septum	Straight, uniform	Deviated
Turbinates	Same as nasal mucosa	
Sinuses	Nontender	Tender
Cranial nerve I	Distinguishes odors	Unable to distinguish odors

Clinical Notes

Intranasal use of cocaine or amphetamines can cause perforation of the nasal septum. Perforation can also be due to surgery or the long-term use of inhaled corticosteroid therapy. Therefore, ask the patient "Have you had nasal surgery?" and "Do you regularly take any medications? What kind, how often do you take them, and for how long have you taken them?"

Pale-blue tinged nasal mucosa with swollen turbinates is characteristic of allergy; red, swollen mucosa is typical of acute infectious rhinitis.

Geriatric Considerations

	Normal Findings
Nose	More prominent because of loss of subcutaneous fat
	Coarse, stiff hairs, protruding from nostrils
Sense of smell	Decreased

Clinical Note

A decreased sense of smell may contribute to decreased food intake and failure to detect the smell of smoke or gas.

Pediatric Considerations

History

Mouth breathing?
Snoring?
Allergic salute?

Hyponasal phonation?
Fetid odor to breath?
Recent trauma?

Procedure

It is necessary to hold the infant's mouth closed while alternately occluding each nostril to test for the patency of the nares.

	Normal Findings	Abnormal Findings
Infant, Child, and Adolescent		Nasal flaring
		Nasal discharge
		Noisy breathing
		Encrusted, excoriated nares
		Crease across nose from frequent rubbing of the nose with the hand because of chronic nasal congestion, pruritus, sneezing, or discharge (allergic salute)

11

Assessment of the Mouth and Throat

HISTORY AND CURRENT STATUS QUESTIONS

Use of dentures?	Upper, lower, full, or partial
Dental problems (e.g., toothache, extractions)?	Type, date of onset, associated symptoms, treatment, current status
Dental examination?	Date of last examination
Bleeding gums?	Date of onset, frequency, site of bleeding, severity, presence of local lesions, tendency to bleed or bruise elsewhere
Soreness of the tongue? Sore throat? Difficulty chewing? Difficulty swallowing?	Date of onset, constant or intermittent, severity, precipitating factors, local lesions, effect on eating patterns, treatment and its effectiveness
Lip or oral lesions?	Type, date of onset, associated symptoms, current status

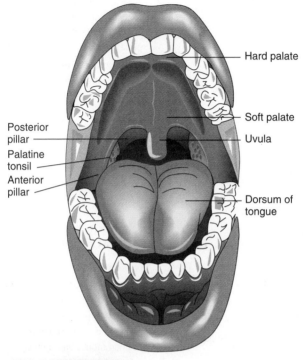

FIGURE 11-1

Anatomy of the mouth and throat.

Voice changes?	Type, date of onset, duration, constant or intermittent, associated or precipitating factors
Oral surgery or injury?	Type, date of occurrence, residual effects
Oral hygiene routines?	Method (e.g., flossing, brushing, toothpaste, mouth rinse), frequency

| Tobacco use? | Type (e.g., cigarettes, cigars, chewing tobacco), how much, how often, for how long (i.e., pack-years). |
| Alcohol use? | Type, pattern of use, amount, for how long |

PHYSICAL EXAMINATION

Equipment

Light
Tongue blade
Clean gloves
Gauze square

Procedures, Techniques, and Findings

Procedure	*Technique*
1. Inspect the lips.	Observe for color, moistness, cracking, ulcers, lumps.
2. Inspect the buccal mucosa.	Ask patient to remove dentures if worn. Direct patient to open mouth and then use a tongue blade and good light to observe for color, pigmentation, ulcers, nodules, or other lesions (Fig. 11–2).
3. Inspect the gums and teeth.	Use tongue blade and light to observe for edema, bleeding, retraction, or discoloration of the gums. Note any missing teeth and the condition of those that remain. Have patient bite down and note alignment of upper and lower jaw.
4. Inspect roof of mouth.	Use tongue blade and light to

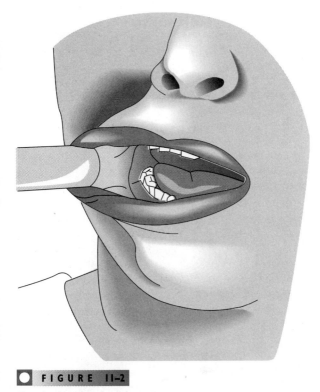

FIGURE 11-2

Examination of the buccal mucosa.

observe the color and structure of the hard palpate.

5. Inspect all the surfaces of the tongue and the floor of the mouth.

Use tongue blade and light to observe tongue for discolored areas, nodules, or ulcerations. Observe dorsum of the tongue for color, surface texture, and pattern of papillae.

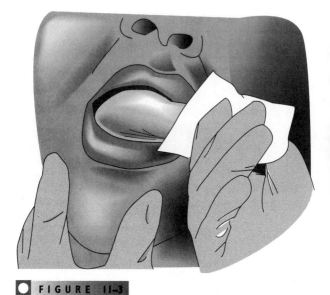

⬤ FIGURE 11-3

Grasping the tongue with a gloved hand and gauze square to inspect its sides.

Ask patient to stick the tongue out. With a gloved right hand grasp the tip of the tongue in a square of gauze and pull it left. Inspect it. Reverse procedure to inspect opposite area of tongue (Fig. 11-3).

Observe the area under the tongue for lesions and check for tenderness.

6. Inspect the structure of the throat.

Ask patient to open mouth. Then depress the middle of the tongue with a tongue blade. Observe for symmetry, color,

7. Test cranial nerve X (vagus nerve, which provides motor innervation to the palate, pharynx, and larynx).		exudate, ulceration, edema, and enlargement of the tonsils. Use tongue blade to depress the tongue. Ask the patient to say "ah" and watch for rise of soft palate.
8. Test cranial nerve XII (hypoglossal nerve, which provides motor innervation to the tongue).		Ask the patient to stick out the tongue and observe for symmetry.

	Normal Findings	Abnormal Findings (Table 11–1)
Lips	Smooth, pink, moist, intact free of lesions Blue tinge due to melanin pigment may be normal in dark-skinned persons	Dryness, cracks, fissures, pallor, cyanosis, drooping, involuntary movements, lesions
Buccal mucosa	Smooth, pink, moist, intact Patchy areas of hyperpigmentation in blacks	Pallor, erythema, cyanosis, edema, bleeding, ulcers, white patches, other lesions
Gums	Pink, moist, intact, clearly defined margins Dark line along gingival margin may be seen in blacks	Dryness, tenderness, edema, bleeding, ulcers, white patches, other lesions
Teeth	32 pearly white and shiny, stable, smooth edges, clean and free of debris	Missing, broken, or loose teeth, cavities, dark brown discoloration

T A B L E 11-1
Common Variations and Abnormalities of the Mouth and Throat

Location	Variation/Abnormality	Description and Significance
Lips	Herpes labialis (cold sore)	Clear vesicles that scab, often located at junction of lips and face; caused by herpes simplex virus; heal in 1–3 weeks
Gums	Hyperplasia	Enlargement of the gums that may impinge onto teeth; associated with puberty, pregnancy, and long-term use of phenytoin; also seen in leukemia
	Gingivitis	*Chronic:* red, swollen gums; may cause pain or bleed on brushing or flossing; often related to poor mouth care or poorly fitting dentures
		Acute: foul taste in mouth, malaise, occasional fever and lymphadenopathy; noncontagious infection
Buccal mucosa	Aphthous ulcer (canker sore)	Shallow pseudomembrane covered ulcer with a ring of erythema; painful; more often seen in women; cause unknown; disappears in 1–2 weeks

Table continued on following page

TABLE 11–1
Common Variations and Abnormalities of the Mouth and Throat *Continued*

Location	Variation/Abnormality	Description and Significance
Buccal mucosa, tongue/lip	Leukoplakia	Areas of chalky white plaque with well-defined borders that are not easily rubbed off; associated with chronic irritation and are precancerous
Tongue	Smooth	Loss of papillae results in a very red, slick shiny appearance; associated with deficiency of vitamin B_{12}, folic acid, niacin, riboflavin, pyridoxine, and iron; accompanied by burning and dryness; also called atrophic glossitis

Table continued on following page

TABLE 11-1
Common Variations and Abnormalities of the Mouth and Throat *Continued*

Location	Variation/Abnormality	Description and Significance
Pharynx	Hypertrophied tonsils	Enlarged tonsils that may reach midline when tongue is protruded; enlargement is not clinically significant
	Pharyngitis	Bright red throat with patches of white or yellow exudate; swollen uvula, sore throat, fever, and large, tender cervical nodes
	Vagal nerve paralysis	Soft palate on affected side does not rise on saying "ah"; uvula deviates to nonaffected side

Table continued on following page

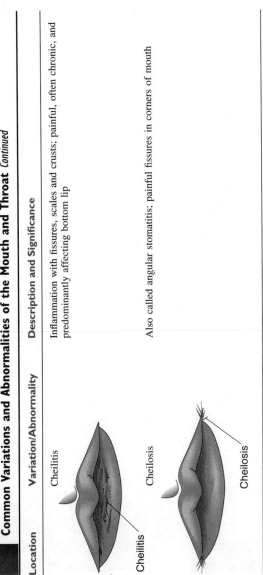

TABLE 11-1
Common Variations and Abnormalities of the Mouth and Throat *Continued*

Location	Variation/Abnormality	Description and Significance
	Cheilitis	Inflammation with fissures, scales and crusts; painful, often chronic, and predominantly affecting bottom lip
	Cheilosis	Also called angular stomatitis; painful fissures in corners of mouth

Cheilitis

Cheilosis

Table continued on following page

TABLE II–I
Common Variations and Abnormalities of the Mouth and Throat *Continued*

Location	Variation/Abnormality	Description and Significance
	Hairy tongue	May be black, brown, or yellow

Table continued on following page

TABLE 11-1
Common Variations and Abnormalities of the Mouth and Throat *Continued*

Location	Variation/Abnormality	Description and Significance
	Geographic tongue	Red shiny areas with raised pearly borders give the appearance of a map that changes every few days; no clinical significance

Table continued on following page

TABLE 11–1
Common Variations and Abnormalities of the Mouth and Throat *Continued*

Location	Variation/Abnormality	Description and Significance
	Fissured tongue	Deep irregular furrows create a scrotal appearance to the dorsum of the tongue; not clinically significant
	Varicose veins	Small, round purple or blue-black swellings on underside of tongue; appear with age and have no clinical significance

Roof of the mouth

Hard palate	Pale, moist, intact	Extreme paleness, erythema
	Bony ridge down the center (torus palatinus) is frequently seen in Asians, Eskimos, and Native Americans (Fig. 11–4)	
Soft palate	Pink, moist, intact	Erythema, pallor

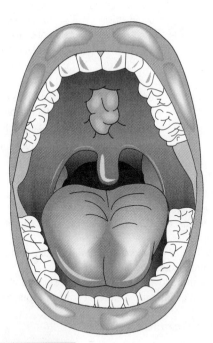

FIGURE 11-4
Torus palatinus.

Tongue	Pink, moist, intact, smooth movement, papillae on dorsal aspect, absence of furrows	Dryness, redness, pallor, white patches, nodules, ulcers, fissures, dehydration furrows on dorsal tongue, asymmetrical contour, jerky or unilateral movement
Throat	Mucosa pink, moist and intact; uvula midline with elevation on phonation; tonsillar pillars symmetrical	Dryness, redness, pallor, white patches, edema, ulcers or other lesions, enlarged tonsils with exudate, deviated uvula, presence of a red or gray membrane
Cranial nerve X	Soft palate rises on "ah"	Soft palate does not rise on "ah"
Cranial nerve XII	Symmetry of protruded tongue	Lateral deviation of protruded tongue

Clinical Notes

Third molars may be normally absent, especially among Asian and white populations.

Oral malignancies are common on the sides and bottom of the tongue.

Bright red areas of mucous membrane under dentures suggest denture sore mouth.

Palpate with a gloved finger any oral lesions to check for thickening or infiltration suggestive of malignancy.

Geriatric Considerations

	Normal Findings
Teeth	May appear uniformly yellowed

	Receding gums with a V-shaped indentation around tooth, giving appearance of being "long in tooth"
Tongue	Smoother than in younger adult because of atrophy of papillae
	Longitudinal and latitudinal fissures may occur
Saliva	Diminished production, resulting in drier appearance of oral cavity
Buccal mucosa	Thinner and shinier than in younger adult

Clinical Note

Remove dentures during examination. Observe for fit and presence of sores or irritations secondary to friction from poorly fitting dentures.

Pediatric Considerations

History

Does child or caretaker brush child's teeth?
Is child under the supervision of a dentist and/or orthodontist?
Fluoridated water, fluoride supplements, dose?
Drinking from a bottle or cup?

Physical Examination

Procedure

When a child resists an examination of the mouth, slide a tongue blade in laterally along the buccal mucosa and insert it behind the molars to induce the gag reflex, which results in an opening of the mouth.

	Normal Findings	*Abnormal Findings*
Infant	Retention cysts on gums	Mouth breathing

	Small calluses on gums and/or lips from vigorous nursing	Thrush: white plaques on oral mucosa that can not be removed
	Epstein's pearls on palate	
	No tonsillar tissue	
	Symmetrical movement of lips, tongue, and palate with sucking	
	Frenulum of tongue varies in thickness; extends to alveolar ridge	
Child and Adolescent	Large tonsils before age 10	
	Symmetry of tonsils and pharyngeal pillars	
	Crypts of tonsils contain concretions and/or food, which appears white	Mouth breathing Fetid breath Dental staining Dental caries Malocclusion
	Geographic tongue	Smooth or cherry-red tongue
		Aphthous ulcers
		Koplik's spots

Clinical Notes

When a child presents with a croupy cough, hoarseness, throat pain, and drooling while sitting upright in order to breathe, *do not examine the oral cavity and pharynx, do not introduce a tongue blade.* These are the signs of epiglottitis, a potentially fatal condition. Examination of the oral cavity may result in complete airway obstruction.

Although there is a timetable for the sequence and eruption of primary teeth there is wide variation in normal children. Without other signs and symptoms there is no need for alarm. A general guide for children under 2 is that the child's age in months minus 6 should equal the number of teeth.

Assessment of the Neck

HISTORY AND CURRENT STATUS QUESTIONS

Injury?	Description, date of occurrence, symptoms, treatment, residual effects
Pain?	Date of onset; constant or intermittent; precipitating movements; associated factors (such as time of day); specific activities (such as long periods of driving, reading, or other close work)
Stiffness or limitation of movement?	Date of onset; constant or intermittent; associated factors (such as time of day); specific activities (such as long periods of driving, reading, or computer use)
Sore throat?	Date of onset, severity (e.g., ability to swallow solids, liquids, saliva), associated symptoms (e.g., cough, upper respiratory tract congestion, fever); precipitating factors

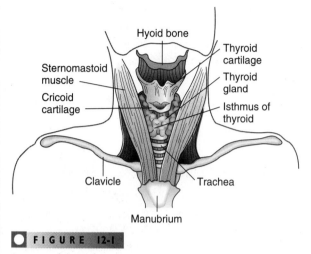

FIGURE 12-1

Anatomy of the neck.

Difficulty swallowing?	Date of onset; acute or gradual onset; constant or intermittent; ability to swallow solids, liquids, and saliva; changes in diet due to dysphagia
Hoarseness?	Acute or chronic; date of onset; constant or intermittent; precipitating factors such as overuse of voice, allergy, smoking, or exposure to other inhaled irritants; associated symptoms (e.g., cough, sore throat, fever)
Lumps or swellings?	Date first noticed, size, location, tenderness, worsened or improved since onset
Thyroid disease/surgery?	Date of occurrence, type, treatment, current medications

Recent weight change?	How much, over what period of time
Change in activity tolerance?	Ask for examples
Temperature intolerance?	Heat or cold

PHYSICAL EXAMINATION

Equipment

Stethoscope

Procedures, Techniques, and Findings

Procedure	*Technique*
1. Inspect the neck for appearance and position.	Observe symmetry and posture with patient sitting up.
2. Check neck movement: flexion, extension, lateral abduction, and rotation.	Direct patient to put head back, put the chin on the chest, touch the chin to each shoulder and bend the right ear to the right shoulder and the left ear to the left shoulder without raising the shoulder.
3. Inspect the carotid artery and jugular vein.	Observe for jugular distention and marked carotid pulsation.
4. Inspect and palpate the trachea for deviation from the midline position. Feel for motion.	Place your index finger along one side of the trachea. Note the space between it and the sternocleidomastoid muscle. Repeat on the other side and compare the spaces (Fig. 12–2).
5. Inspect the neck for the thyroid gland.	Direct patient to lift the chin and observe for the thyroid. Ask patient to take a sip from a glass of water, lift chin, and swallow. Observe for movement of the thyroid and if

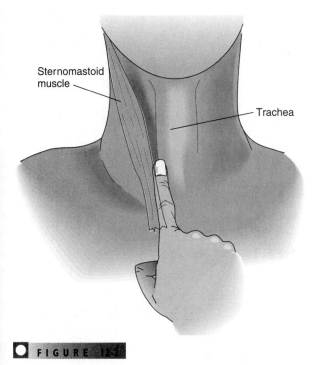

Sternomastoid
muscle

Trachea

FIGURE 12-2

Palpation of the trachea for deviation.

seen note its contour and
symmetry.

6. Palpate the thyroid for size,
   shape, and consistency.

Stand behind the patient and
ask the patient to put the head
back slightly. Place fingers of
both hands on the patient's
neck with the index fingers just
below the cricoid cartilage
(*Fig. 12–3*). Ask the patient to
swallow and feel for the rise of
the thyroid isthmus under your

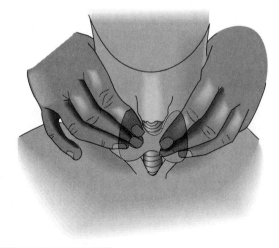

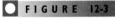

FIGURE 12-3

Position for palpation of the thyroid.

7. Auscultate any enlarged thyroid for vascular sounds.

8. Palpate for cervical lymph nodes.

fingers. Move fingers down and to the sides to feel any palpable parts of the lateral lobes.

Place bell stethoscope over lateral lobes and listen.

Using pads of first two fingers palpate both sides of the neck simultaneously. Use light to moderate pressure and move the skin over the underlying tissues rather than moving your fingers to each area. Begin in front of the ear and progress as shown in Table 12–1. To examine the submental node, palpate with one hand and place the other on

T A B L E 12–1
Pattern of Palpation of Cervical Nodes

Node	Location
1. Preauricular	In front of ear
2. Posterior auricular	Over the mastoid process in back of the ear
3. Occipital	At the posterior base of the skull
4. Tonsillar	At the mandibular angle
5. Submaxillary	Midpoint between the mandibular angle and the tip of the mandible
6. Submental	Midline behind the tip of the mandible
7. Superficial cervical	Over the sternocleidomastoid muscle
8. Posterior cervical	Along the anterior margin of the trapezius muscle
9. Deep cervical	Deep to the sternocleidomastoid muscle
10. Supraclavicular	Deep in angle of the clavicle and sternocleidomastoid muscle

1. Anterior auricular
2. Posterior auricular
3. Occipital
4. Tonsillar
5. Submaxillary
6. Submental
7. Superficial cervical
8. Posterior cervical
9. Deep cervical
10. Supraclavicular

top of the patient's head for
support.

	Normal Findings	*Abnormal Findings*
Neck		
Appearance	Symmetrical Proportional to head and shoulders	Unusual shortness, asymmetry, fullness, edema, masses, scars
Movement	From upright position: Flexion 45 degrees Extension 55 degrees Lateral abduction 40 degrees Rotation 70 degrees	Less than the normal range of motion
	Coordinated, controlled movement	Uncoordinated or uncontrolled movement
Jugular vein		Distended
Carotid artery	Mild pulsations	Marked pulsations
Trachea	Midline, nontender, distinct rings	Lateral deviation, tender, edematous
Thyroid	Usually not visible, smooth, symmetrical, and rubbery on palpation	Visible enlargement, nodular, tender, bruit
Cervical lymph nodes	Not palpable or ≤1 cm, smooth, firm, mobile, nontender with definite margins	Palpable Inflamed: tender, mobile, indefinite margins Malignant: nontender, fixed,

hard, nodular, ir-
regular shape,
indefinite
margins

Geriatric Considerations

Normal Findings

Submandibular salivary glands	Prolapsed and palpable as soft masses bilaterally in upper neck, below jaw
Length of neck	Shortened because of muscle atrophy and loss of fat

Clinical Note

Perform range of motion of the neck slowly, as the older patient may experience dizziness with side movements.

Pediatric Considerations

	Normal Findings	*Abnormal Findings*
Infant	Thyroglossal duct cyst midline over trachea	Short or webbed neck indicative of genetic syndrome
Infant and Child, and Adolescent	Full flexion	Nuchal rigidity: limited flexion indicative of meningeal irritation
	Resistance to full flexion	Suprasternal retractions indicative of upper airway obstruction
		Torticollis: head tilted toward injured sternocleidomastoid muscle; firm mass palpated in muscle

13

Assessment of the Breasts and Axillae

HISTORY AND CURRENT STATUS QUESTIONS

Personal history of breast disease?

History of cancer, tumors, cysts, mastitis, galactorrhea, trauma, breast surgery (mastectomy, lumpectomy, biopsies, implants, or other cosmetic or reconstructive surgery), date(s) of occurrence, treatment, and outcome

Family history of breast disease?

Type of disease; age at onset; relationship of the affected person to the patient, noting maternal or paternal side as appropriate; treatment, and outcome

Breast examinations?

Frequency of breast self-examination and date last performed; frequency and date of last professional breast examination

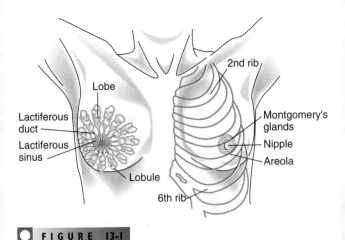

FIGURE 13-1

Anatomy of the breast.

Mammogram?	Frequency of mammograms; date and results of last mammogram
Lumps?	Location, date discovered, tender or nontender, any noticeable change in size, any relationship to menstruation
Tenderness/pain?	Localized or diffuse; unilateral or bilateral; constant or intermittent; severity; precipitating, aggravating, or relieving factors
Swelling?	Date of onset, relationship to menses, unilateral or bilateral
Skin changes?	Type, venous prominence, location, onset, sores, discolorations
Nipple discharge?	Unilateral or bilateral, color, amount, odor, frequency, associated factors and symptoms

Axillary lumps?	Location, date discovered, change in size since discovery, change related to the menstrual cycle
Axillary tenderness?	Date of onset, location, severity, precipitating and/or aggravating factors, relationship to menstruation
Axillary rash?	Date of onset, unilateral or bilateral, associated symptoms such as pruritus or burning, change in hygienic products, other potential precipitating factors

PHYSICAL EXAMINATION

Equipment

Small pillow
Sheet
Towel or gown for draping

Procedures, Techniques, and Findings

Procedure	*Technique*
1. Inspect the breasts for size, color, venous pattern, skin appearance, vascularity, contour, and symmetry.	Begin the examination with the patient in a sitting position with arms at her sides (Fig. 13–2A).
2. Inspect the areolae for shape, color, hair, and masses.	Continue to inspect the breasts while the patient raises her arms over her head, lowers them, presses her hands against her hips, and, if breasts are large and pendulous, leans forward (Fig. 13–2 B–D).
3. Observe the nipples for size, shape, symmetry, and direction in which they point.	
4. Inspect the axillae for hair distribution, cleanliness, uniformity, and skin condition.	

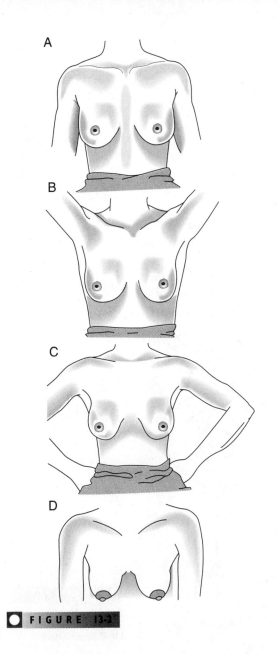

FIGURE 13-2

5. Palpate each breast, including the tail of Spence, noting masses, consistency, tenderness, and lymph nodes.

With patient sitting, hands at sides, use the pads of your fingers and a firm circular motion to move the skin over the breast tissue. Proceed with palpation following a specific pattern such as spiraling out from the nipple, tracing the spokes of a wheel, or following vertical or horizontal lines (Fig. 13–3).

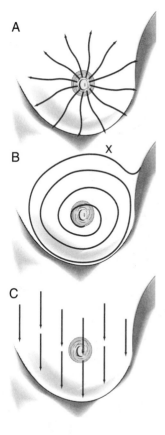

A

B

X

C

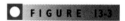

● FIGURE 13-3

Patterns of breast palpation. *A*, Spokes of a wheel. *B*, Spiral. *C*, Vertical lines.

D

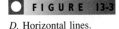

FIGURE 13-3 *Continued*

D, Horizontal lines.

Examine each quadrant and the tail of the breast. Next, repeat the palpation with the patient lying on her back with her arm (on the side being palpated) placed behind her head, and a small pillow under side to be palpated (Fig. 13–4).

Compare the breasts to each other. If the patient reports a problem in one breast, palpate the other breast first to establish a baseline assessment, then palpate the affected breast and attempt to locate the lump or tenderness.

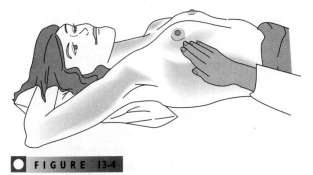

FIGURE 13-4

Recumbent position for breast palpation.

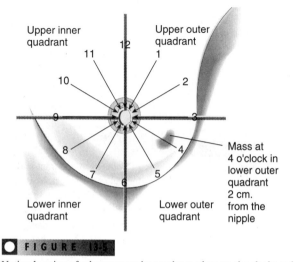

Upper inner quadrant

Upper outer quadrant

12
11
1
10
2
9
3
8
4
7
5
6

Mass at 4 o'clock in lower outer quadrant 2 cm. from the nipple

Lower inner quadrant

Lower outer quadrant

● FIGURE 13-5

Noting location of a breast mass by quadrant, place on the clock, and distance from the nipple.

	Verify its position with the patient when found. If a lump is felt, describe the size, consistency, shape, boundaries, mobility, tenderness, and location, noting quadrant, distance from nipple, and place on the clock (Fig. 13–5).
6. Check for nipple discharge.	Gently compress each nipple and note whether there is any discharge (Fig. 13–6). Note color, consistency, quantity, odor, presence of blood tinge or streak in *any* discharge present.
7. Palpate the axillae.	Ask the patient to sit and relax the arm on the side to be examined, letting it "hang down."

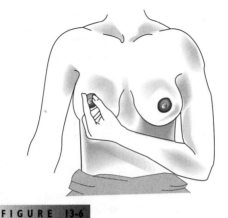

FIGURE 13-6

Nipple compression to check for discharge.

Use your right hand to examine the left axilla and vice versa. Use your opposite hand to support the patient's arm (Fig. 13–7).

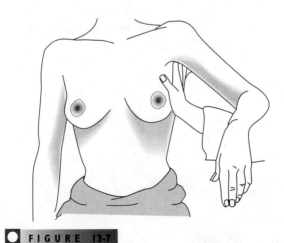

FIGURE 13-7

Position for palpation of the axilla.

With your fingers together and slightly cupped, reach as high into the axilla as possible.

Press inward toward the chest wall and move your fingers firmly downward to check for central nodes.

Repeat the maneuver, moving your fingers down the anterior border of the axilla to check for pectoral (anterior) nodes and along the inner aspect of the upper arm to check for lateral nodes.

Step behind the patient and repeat the maneuver, moving fingers down the posterior border of the axilla to check for posterior nodes.

Check infraclavicular nodes if enlarged or tender axillary nodes are found (Fig. 13–8).

Repeat for the opposite side.

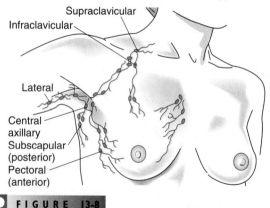

Supraclavicular
Infraclavicular
Lateral
Central axillary
Subscapular (posterior)
Pectoral (anterior)

FIGURE 13-8

Location of lymph node groups draining the breast.

	Normal Findings	**Abnormal Findings**
Size and symmetry	Symmetrical, one breast may be slightly larger	Asymmetrical, marked difference in size
Contour	Conical to pendulous	Retraction, dimpling, flattening, or other marked difference (Fig. 13–9*A*)
Color	Similar to normal skin on the trunk; striae often follow pregnancy.	Erythema or other discoloration
Venous pattern	Faint, symmetrical	Asymmetrical dilation (Fig. 13–9*B*)

A Retraction, dimpling

B Venous prominence

◯ FIGURE 13-9

Observable breast abnormalities. *A,* Dimpling. *B,* Venous prominence.
Illustration continued on following page

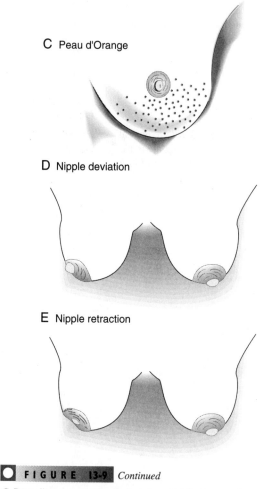

C, Peau d'orange. *D*, Nipple deviation. *E*, Nipple retraction.

| Skin appearance | Smooth, soft | Peau d 'orange (orange peel) appearance, lesions (Fig. 13–9*C*) |

Consistency	Uniformly loose to dense	Thickening, masses
	Feels firm to soft, smooth, elastic	
Tenderness	Tender if pre-menstrual	Tender or painful
Masses	None	Palpable mass, feels like the tip of the nose or harder
Nipples and areolae	No discharge	Discharge, retraction, deviation, recent inversion (Fig. 13–9D–E)
	Symmetrical	
Axillae	Occasionally one or more soft, nontender central nodes; otherwise not usually palpable	Palpable nodes

Clinical Notes

For men, inspect and palpate breasts in sitting position only.

Geriatric Considerations
Physical Examination

	Normal Findings
Female breasts	Fine glandular texture due to a replacement of glandular tissue with fatty tissue
	Elongated, flat breasts as suspensory ligaments relax
Nipples	Ducts surrounding the nipple are easily palpated as firm stringy strands
	Nipples may be retracted but can be pulled out
Axillae	Sparse, gray hair

TABLE 13-1
Characteristics of Benign and Malignant Breast Lumps

	Benign Cyst	Benign Fibroadenoma	Breast Cancer
Age at occurrence	30 to menopause, after which regression occurs	Puberty to 55	30 and over, with great incidence in the middle-aged and elderly
Number	Single or multiple	Usually multiple, sometimes single	Single
Shape	Round	Round, oval, or lobed	Irregular
Consistency	Soft to firm and rubbery	Usually firm	Hard
Delieeation	Clearly defined edges	Clearly defined edges	Poorly defined edges
Mobility	Mobile	Mobile	Fixed
Tenderness	Often tender, especially premenstrually	Usually nontender	Usually nontender
Retraction signs			
Abnormal count	Absent	Absent	Often present
Dimpling	Absent	Absent	Often present
Nipple retraction or deviation	Absent	Absent	Often present
Peaud 'orange skin	Absent	Absent	Often present
Increased venous prominence	Absent	Absent	Often present

Clinical Note

Breast cancer risk increases with age. Because of the time in which they were raised, older women often find it difficult to examine their own breasts. Take time to teach breast self-examination and the need for routine mammography.

Pediatric Considerations

History

Taking any substance including OTC medications, "herbal" or "homeopathic" remedies?

Age of thelarche (the beginning of breast development at puberty)?

Age of menarche (the appearance of the first menstrual period)?

Explore areas related to sexual precocity and sexual abuse.

Physical Examination

Note Tanner stage:

Tanner I: No breast development

Tanner II: Breast bud (possible asymmetry of development with tenderness)

Tanner III: Areolae and breast tissue enlarge

Tanner IV: Areolae and papillae form own contour

Tanner V: Full adult maturity

	Normal Findings	Abnormal Findings
Newborn	Supernumerary nipples	
	Leakage of milklike substance from nipples	
Infant	Palpable breast tissue	Persistent breast tissue beyond infancy; enlarging breast buds

Adolescent	Thelarche during preteen years	
	Thelarche at 9 years	Thelarche at <8 years
	Gynecomastia in males	Gynecomastia in males that does not subside with advancing maturity

Clinical Notes

Be sensitive to embarrassment and self-consciousness in the adolescent.

14

Assessment of the Chest and Lungs

HISTORY AND CURRENT STATUS QUESTIONS

Personal history   History of cardiovascular disease, such as an enlarged heart, abnormal cardiac rhythm, septal or valvular defects,

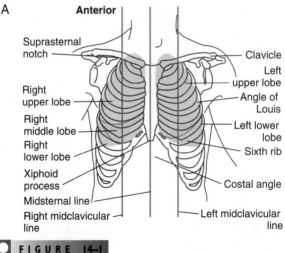

A   **Anterior**

Suprasternal notch

Clavicle

Left upper lobe

Right upper lobe

Angle of Louis

Right middle lobe

Left lower lobe

Right lower lobe

Sixth rib

Xiphoid process

Costal angle

Midsternal line

Right midclavicular line

Left midclavicular line

FIGURE 14–1

Thoracic landmarks. *A*, Anterior chest.

Illustration continued on following page

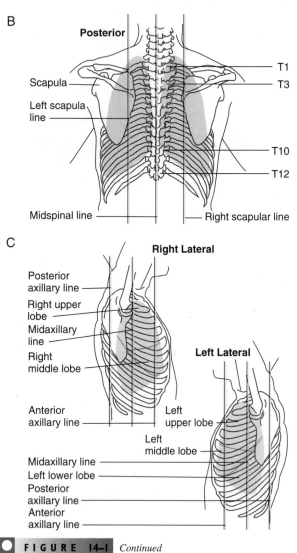

O FIGURE 14–1 *Continued*

B, Posterior chest. *C*, Right lateral and left lateral chest.

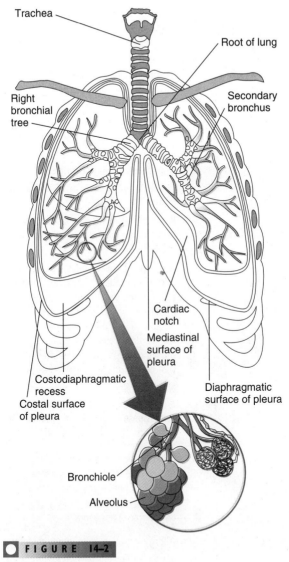

Anatomy of the lungs.

coronary artery disease, congestive heart failure, angina or myocardial infarction

History of pulmonary disease, such as asthma, tuberculosis, pneumonia, bronchitis, chronic obstructive pulmonary disease (COPD), sarcoidosis, or lung cancer

Any recent or remote trauma to the chest or thorax?

Abnormalities of or arthritic conditions involving the spine, ribs, scapula, clavicle, or sternum

Frequent muscle spasms, or at risk for occupational or recreational overuse injuries

Note age of onset, specific problem, treatment rendered (including diagnostic tests and procedures, surgery, medications, and current status

Family history

Any cardiovascular, pulmonary, or musculoskeletal problems affecting the thorax or lungs as described above

Note the relation to the patient, specific problem, age of onset, age of death, and disease or problem responsible for the death of the family member

Tobacco?

If patient or family members smoke, record type (cigarettes, cigars, pipe), how long, how many cigarettes or packs per day, for how many years (written as "pack-years")

Allergies?

Allergy to pollen, dust, other airborne irritants, medicines, drugs, food, chemicals

Chest pain?

Constant or intermittent, pleuritic or nonpleuritic, localized or diffuse; provocative/palliative influences, quality, region, severity and timing (PQRST) (see Fig. 15–2 in Chap. 15).

Palpitations?

Time of occurrence (with exertion, at rest), previous ECG or Holter monitoring

Shortness of breath?

Time of occurrence (with exertion or at rest), change in respiratory rate and rhythm; evidence of a change in mental status, use of accessory muscles to breathe, cyanosis, clubbing of nails, or shift of the trachea

Cough?

Type (hacking, constant, intermittent, or rare), time of occurrence (early morning), evokes chest pain, productive or nonproductive; Color and consistency of the sputum (thick, thin, clear, yellow, green, blood streaked); cultures, results

Hemoptysis?

Blood-streaked sputum or frank blood, amount (a teaspoon, a cup), duration

Associated symptoms?

Fever, chills, night sweats, nausea, vomiting, diarrhea, fatigue, malaise, weight loss, headache, dizziness, syncope, and diaphoresis

Occupational risks?

Exposure to asbestos, pollutants, chemicals, radiation, vapors and fumes

Medications?

Some medications may cause the symptoms above as side effects

Past work-up?

Chest x-ray, pulmonary function tests, arterial blood gas, lumbar sacral spine or rib film, ECG, echocardiogram,

Holter monitor, exercise tolerance test, or cardiac catheterization

Vaccines?   Tuberculosis purified protein derivative (PPD), influenza, pneumonia

PHYSICAL EXAMINATION

Equipment

Stethoscope
Tape measure

Procedures, Techniques, and Findings

Procedure	*Technique*
1. Prepare the patient for the examination.	Ask the patient to undress and sit up on the examining table. Observe the posterior thorax from a midline position behind the patient. Observe the anterior thorax with the patient lying supine.
2. Inspect and palpate the skin and nails for color, lesions, turgor, and abnormalities.	Refer to Chapter 6, Assessment of the Skin, Hair, and Nails.
3. Inspect and palpate the thorax, clavicles, scapulas, ribs, and spine for contour and abnormalities (Fig. 14–3). Note any congenital anomalies, traumatic injury, postsurgical alterations, masses, lesions, tenderness or abnormal slopes or contours.	Inspect as described above. Ask the patient to bend over at the waist to further inspect the curvature of the spine. Palpate and compare symmetrical areas of the posterior and anterior thorax using your fingertips or the "ball" of your hand (posterior palm) (Figs. 14–4, 14–5).

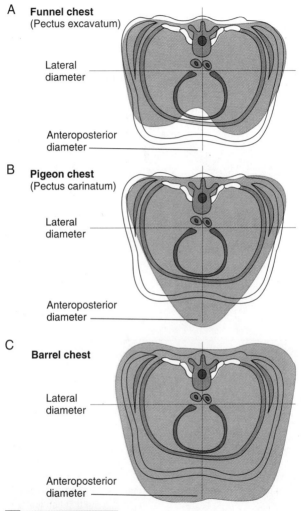

A **Funnel chest**
(Pectus excavatum)

Lateral diameter

Anteroposterior diameter

B **Pigeon chest**
(Pectus carinatum)

Lateral diameter

Anteroposterior diameter

C **Barrel chest**

Lateral diameter

Anteroposterior diameter

FIGURE 14–3

Common chest deformities. *A,* Funnel chest. *B,* Pigeon chest. *C,* Barrel chest.

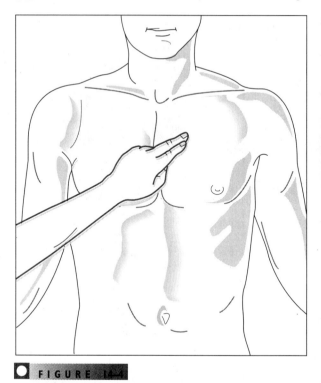

FIGURE 14-4

Palpation of the thorax using fingertips.

4. Inspect the patient's pattern of breathing; note abnormalities of rate or rhythm (Fig. 14–6B).

Attempt to observe the patient without making him aware that you are observing his respirations. A good technique is to pretend that you are taking the patient's pulse, while you are actually observing his respiratory pattern.

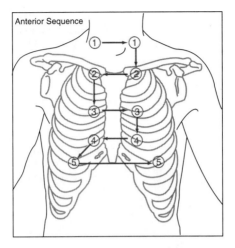

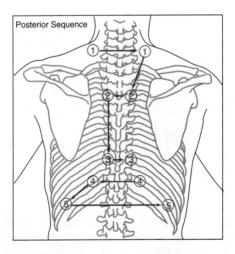

FIGURE 14-5

Compare symmetrical areas of posterior and anterior thorax.

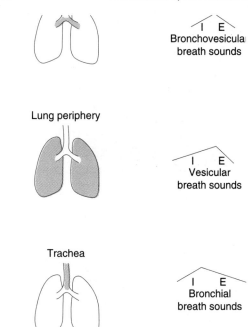

A, Breath sounds. I = inspiration E = Expiration *Figure cont.*

5. Inspect and palpate the patient's breasts and axillae for shape, contour, symmetry, lesions, masses, dimpling, vasculature, and discharge.

Refer to Chapter 13, Assessment of the Breasts and Axillae.

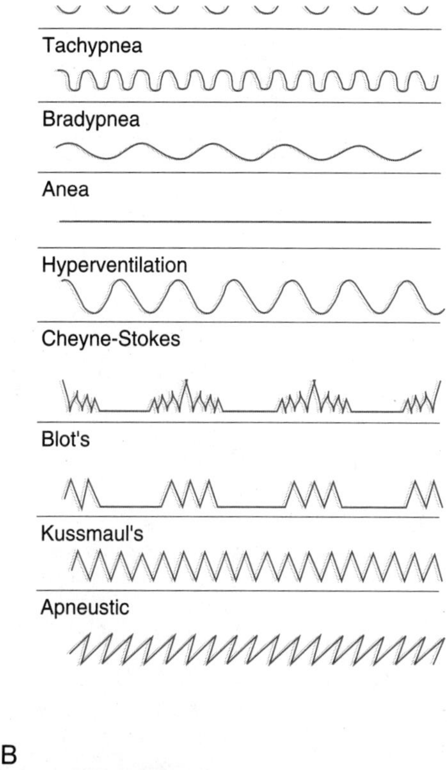

Tachypnea

Bradypnea

Anea

Hyperventilation

Cheyne-Stokes

Blot's

Kussmaul's

Apneustic

B

FIGURE 14–6 CONT.

B, Respiratory patterns.

6. Palpate for tactile fremitus (Fig. 14–7).	Ask the patient to say "99," "99," "99" as you place the "ball" (the area of the posterior palm near the proximal finger joints) of one hand on

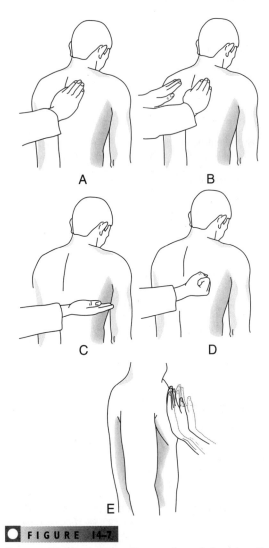

● FIGURE 14-7

Thorax palpation. *A,* Use palmar surface of fingertips. *B,* Apply fingertips of both hands simultaneously. *C,* Use ulnar aspect of the hand. *D,* Use ulnar aspect of the closed fist. *E,* Place open hands simultaneously on chest.

each of the target areas as diagrammed. Compare the transmission of the patient's voice through the chest wall in symmetrical areas (Fig. 14–8).

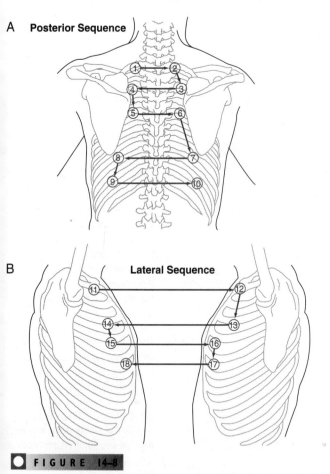

A **Posterior Sequence**

B **Lateral Sequence**

● FIGURE 14-8

Palpate for tactile fremitis. *A*, Posterior sequence. *B*, Lateral sequence. *Figure cont.*

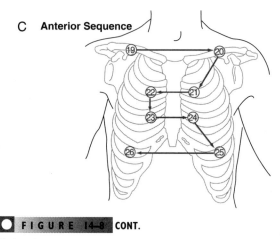

C, Anterior sequence.

FIGURE 14-8 CONT.

| 7. Palpate for respiratory excursion. | Stand behind the patient with your thumbs placed on the spinal processes at the level of the tenth ribs. Spread your fingers apart over the lateral thorax [your thumbs pointing toward each other and your fingers pointing away from each other (Fig. 14–9)]. Press your palms inward toward the spine, moving your thumbs closer together with only a small skinfold between them. Now ask the patient to exhale and then take a deep breath and hold it. Observe the movement of your thumbs and note the expanded distance between them. |
| 8. Percuss the posterior and anterior thorax; the quality | To obtain a "percussion" note, press the middle finger of |

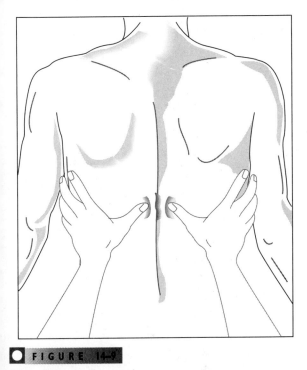

FIGURE 14-9

Palpate for respiratory excursion.

of the "percussion notes" will reveal the nature of underlying tissue.

your left hand firmly on the surface. Cock the middle finger of your right hand and strike the middle finger of your left hand between the distal joint and the fingernail (see Chapter 2, Fig. 2–3). Work your way down the posterior and then the anterior thorax as diagrammed (Fig. 14–10), striking twice in each of the percussion target areas shown;

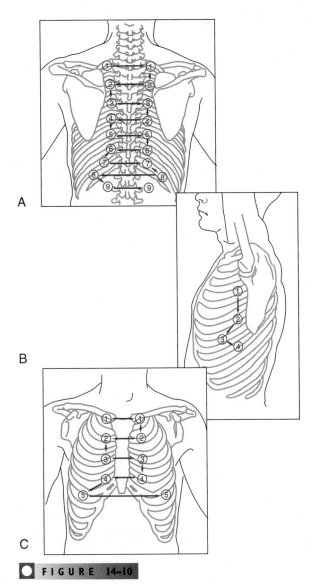

FIGURE 14-10

Thoracic percussion. *A*, Posterior sequence. *B*, Left lateral sequence. *C*, Anterior sequence.

listen for dullness, resonance, or tympany. Dullness will be heard over solid or fluid-filled tissue, resonance over air-filled tissue, and tympany over air-containing tissue that is hyper-inflated (such as the gastric air bubble) (Fig. 14–11).

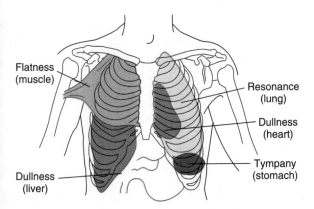

Flatness (muscle)

Dullness (liver)

Resonance (lung)

Dullness (heart)

Tympany (stomach)

Percussion Note	Intensity	Pitch	Duration	Location Example	Disease Entity
Flatness	soft	high	short	thigh	large pleural effusion
Dullness	medium	medium	medium	liver	lobar pneumonia
Resonance	loud	low	long	lung	bronchitis
Hyper-resonance	very loud	lower	longer	none	emphysema pneumo-thorax
Tympany	loud	high	N/A	gastric air bubble	large pneumo-thorax

FIGURE 14–11

Precuss to assess the nature of underlying tissue.

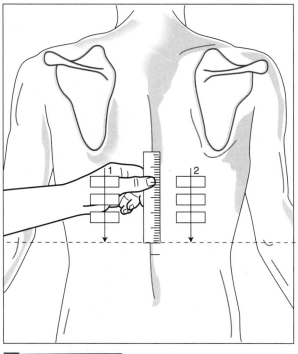

● F I G U R E   14–12

Precuss to assess diaphragmatic excursion. Measure the distance between the point where dullness is initially heard and where diaphragmatic dullness is initially heard.

9. Percuss the diaphragmatic excursion.	Ask the patient to exhale and hold it. Percuss downward from a point of resonance to-ward the diaphragm. Mark the point where dullness is initially heard. Ask the patient to then inhale and hold it. Again percuss downward from a

	point of resonance to the area where diaphragmatic dullness is initially heard. Mark this point and measure the distance between both points (Fig. 14–12).
10. Auscultate the posterior and then the anterior thorax in the fashion diagrammed.	Sit the patient up for both posterior and anterior chest auscultation, since abnormal findings may be masked in a supine patient. With the diaphragm of the stethoscope listen to the patient breathing. Move across and down both the posterior and then the anterior chest in the fashion diagrammed (Fig. 14–13). Discern whether artefactual sounds are occurring and eliminate them before proceeding. Further assess the rate and rhythm of the patient's breathing (see Fig. 14–6*B*.) Identify and distinguish vesicular, bronchovesicular, and bronchial breath sounds from artefactual and adventitious sounds (Figs. 14–14, 14–15). Note any adventitious sounds (Fig. 14–16), their timing (inspiratory or expiratory) and location, and whether they clear with coughing, deep breathing, or position changes

Text continued on page 258

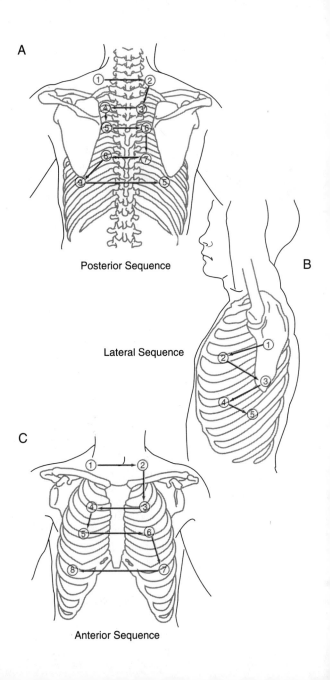

A

Posterior Sequence

B

Lateral Sequence

C

Anterior Sequence

Characteristics of Breath Sounds

Type	Duration	Intensity	Pitch	Location
Vesicular	Insp>Exp	soft	low	most of both lungs
Bronch-vesicular	Insp=Exp	medium	medium	1st and 2nd interspaces anteriorly and between scapula
Bronchial	Insp<Esp	loud	high	Over manubrium if heard at all
Tracheal	Insp<Exp	very loud	high	Over trachea in neck

Ratio of inspiration to expiration

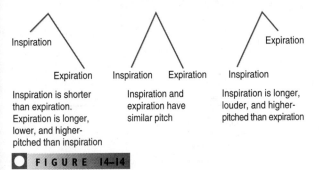

Inspiration is shorter than expiration. Expiration is longer, lower, and higher-pitched than inspiration

Inspiration and expiration have similar pitch

Inspiration is longer, louder, and higher-pitched than expiration

⬤ FIGURE 14-14

Identify breath sounds and rate of inspiration to expiration.

◀ **⬤ FIGURE 14-13**

Auscultate the thorax. *A,* Posterior sequence. *B,* Lateral sequence. *C,* Anterior sequence.

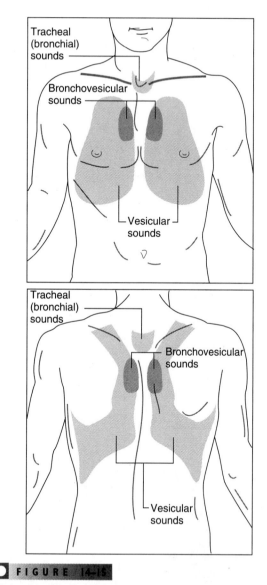

Tracheal
(bronchial)
sounds

Bronchovesicular
sounds

Vesicular
sounds

Tracheal
(bronchial)
sounds

Bronchovesicular
sounds

Vesicular
sounds

FIGURE 14-15

Distinguish vesicular, bronchovesicular, and bronchial breath sounds from artefactual and adventitious sounds.

Sound	Site auscultated	Cause	Description
Crackles (previously called rales)	Most common in dependent lobes: right and left lung bases	Random, sudden reinflation of groups of alveoli; commonly caused by congestive heart failure, pneumonia, and atelectasis	Fine, short, interrupted crackling sounds heard during inspiration, expiration, or both; Vary in pitch: high or low; may or may not change with coughing
Gurgles (previously called rhonchi)	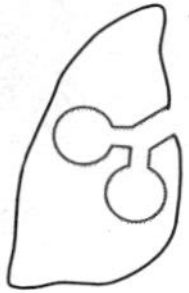 Primarily over trachea and bronchia If loud enough, can be heard over most lung fields	Fluid or mucus in larger airways, causing turbulence	Low-pitched, continuous musical sounds heard more during expiration May be cleared by coughing
Wheezes	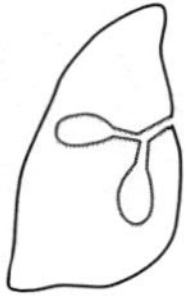 All lung fields	Severely narrowed bronchus	High-pitched, continuous musical sounds heard during inspiration or expiration Do not clear with coughing
Pleural friction rub	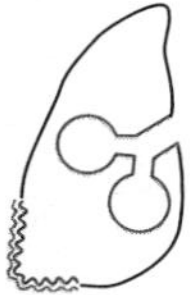 Anterior lateral lung field (if client sitting upright)	Pleura becomes inflamed; parietal pleura rubs against visceral pleura	Has grating quality Heard best during inspiration Does not clear with coughing

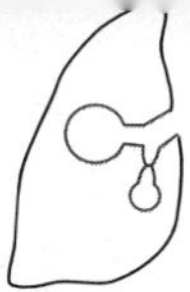

● **FIGURE 14-16**

Note adventitious sounds.

	Normal Findings	Abnormal Findings
Skin and nails	Refer to Chapter 6	Refer to Chapter 6
Thorax	Normal contour (ratio of anterioposterior diameter to lateral diameter equivalent to 1:2 to 5:7)	Barrel chest, funnel chest, pigeon chest, other congenital anomalies, traumatic injury, surgical alterations (see Fig. 14–3)
Ribs	Normal sloping of the ribs	Ribs acquire more of a horizontal slope in emphysema
		Missing ribs or abnormal contour or shape secondary to surgery or trauma
Spine	Straight, without lesions or masses	Abnormal curvatures of the spine (kyphosis, scoliosis), cysts, masses, spina bifida, or incomplete closure of the spine
Breathing	Regular rate between 16 and 20 breaths per minute; regular rhythm where inspiration is approximately equivalent to expiration in length	Tachypnea, bradypnea, hyperpnea, sighing, hyperventilation, ataxia, apnea, Cheyne–Stokes, Kussmaul, wheezing, whistling, respiratory lag, prolonged expiration, bulging

Condition	Auscultation	Percussion	Tactile Fremitus	Vocal Fremitus	Diaphragmatic Excursion	Trachea Position
Normal lung 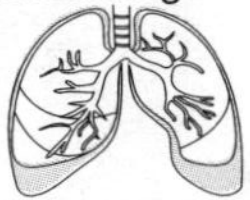	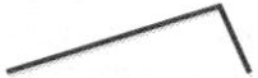 Vesicular breath sounds. No adventitious sounds	Resonant	Present and normal	Normal	3 - 5 cm	Midline
Asthma 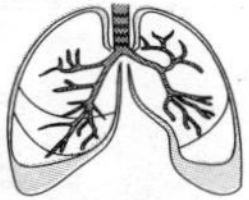	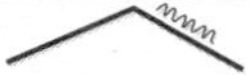 Bronchovesicular breath sounds. Wheezes or Sibilant Rhonchi are usually present.	Hyperresonant	Decreased	Decreased	Normal to slightly decreased	Midline
Atelectasis 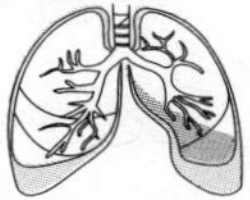	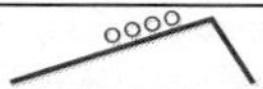 Vesicular breath sounds. Rales may be heard in late inspiration.	Dull to flat over the portion of collapsed lung. Hyperresonant over remaining unaffected portion of the lung.	Decreased or absent	Decreased or absent over affected side	Decreased on affected side	Shifted towards the affected side
Bronchitis 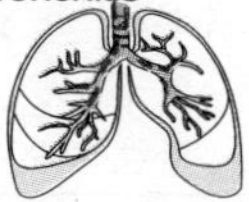	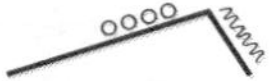 Vesicular breath sounds. Rales and Sibilant Rhonchi present.	Resonant	Normal or increased	Normal	Normal	Midline

FIGURE 14–17 Abnormal lung conditions.

Illustration continued on following page

Condition	Auscultation	Percussion	Tactile Fremitus	Vocal Fremitus	Diaphragmatic Excursion	Trachea Position
Brochiectasis 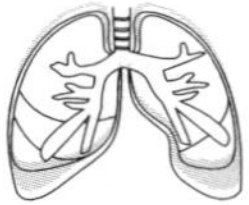	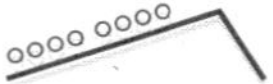 Vesicular breath sounds. Rales may be present.	Resonant or dull	Increased	Normal	Decreased on affected side.	Midline or deviated toward affected side
Emphysema 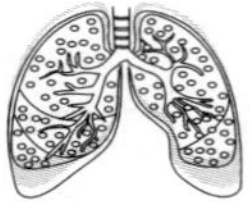	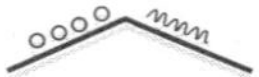 Bronchial breath sounds with prolonged expiration and decreased intensity. Fine rales are often present in late inspiration and occasional rhonchi may be heard.	Resonant to Hyperresonant	Decreased	Normal to decreased	Decreased	Midline
Pleural Effusion 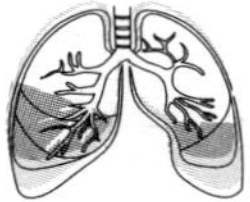	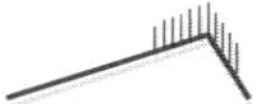 Decreased or absent breath sounds. A pleural friction rub may be heard	Dull to flat	Decreased or absent	Decreased or absent. May have brochophony, egophony, and whispered pectoriloquy if the effusion compresses the lung	Decreased on affected side.	Deviation toward the normal side

FIGURE 14–17 Continued Abnormal lung conditions. Illustration continued on following page

Condition	Auscultation	Percussion	Tactile Fremitus	Vocal Fremitus	Diaphragmatic Excursion	Trachea Position
Pneumonia and consolidation 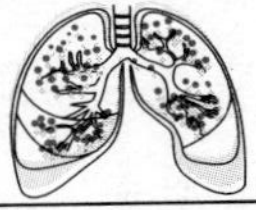	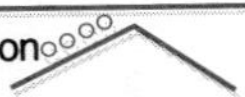 Bronchovesicular or bronchial breath sounds over the affected area. Rales may be present on late inspiration	Dull to flat	Usually increased	Usually increased bronchophony, egophony, and whispered pectoriloquy.	May be decreased on the affected side	Midline
Pneumothorax 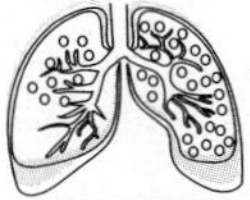	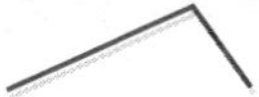 Decreased or absent breath sound. No adventitious sounds present.	Hyperresonant	Absent	Decreased or absent	Decreased on the affected side	Shifted toward the unaffected side
Pulmonary Fibrosis 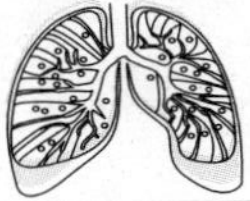	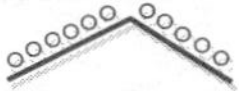 Decreased or absent bronchovesicular sounds. Rales may be heard on inspiration and expiration	Resonant to dull	Usually increased	Increased, Increased whispered pectoriloquy may be present	Decreased	Shifted toward the affected side
Tumor 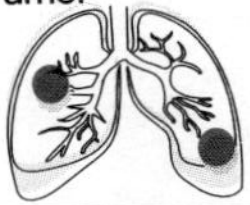	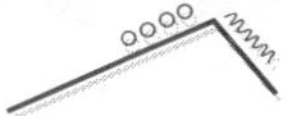 Decreased or absent breath sounds	Dull over mass	Usually increased over mass	Usually increased over mass	Decreased	May be shifted toward unaffected side as a result of extrinsic pressure from the mass

Continued

● FIGURE 14-17   Abnormal lung conditions.

		of the intercostal spaces, use of accessory muscles (see Fig. 14–6)
Breasts	Refer to Chapter 13	Refer to Chapter 13
Muscles	Normal tone, non-tender	Tight spasm, tenderness, atrophy, torn or weakened (as in ventral hernia), masses
Tactile fremitus	Should be equivalent in symmetrical areas overlying lung spaces	Decreased with a soft voice, laryngeal disease or obstruction, COPD, obstructed bronchus, effusion (fluid), fibrosis (thickening), pneumothorax (air), or infiltrating tumor; increased with increased transmission as in consolidated lung (lobar pneumonia)
Respiratory excursion	Normal respiratory excursion will separate the thumbs by 1¼ to 2 inches (see Fig. 14–9)	Limited respiratory excursion may occur with chronic fibrotic disease of the lungs, COPD, emphysema, pulmonary tumors (such as an abdominal mass), or superficial pain
Percussion	Resonance is heard over air-containing	Dullness replaces resonance when

tissue and heard over most of the lung spaces; dullness is heard over fluid-filled or solid tissue and is heard normally over large underlying organs such as the liver and heart; tympany is normal heard over the gastric air bubble in the left upper quadrant

fluid-filled or solid tissue replaces air-containing tissue or occupies the pleural space; this occurs with pleural effusion, lobar pneumonia, abscess, blood (hemothorax), pus (empyema), and infiltration by fibrous tissue or tumor; hyperresonance is heard over hyperinflated lungs, such as in emphysema, or asthma; unilateral hyperresonance suggests pneumothorax or air-filled bulla in the lung (see Fig. 14–11)

Diaphragmatic excursion

Diaphragm descends 3 to 6 cm.

Diaphragm descends <3 cm or >6 cm (see Fig. 14–12)

Auscultation

Artefactual sounds

Normally no artefactual sounds should be heard or this will greatly confuse your results

Identify and remove all artefactual sounds such as those made inadvertently from clothing, muscle contractions, paper, scratching, examiner's fingers on stethoscope or chest

Breath sounds

Breath sounds should normally sound symmetrical; inspiration should be approximately equivalent to expiration in duration; adventitious sounds should be absent (see Figs. 14–14, 14–15)

A few individuals will normally have fine crackles present in their bilateral lung bases; otherwise, there should be no crackles, wheezes, or rubs audible

Longer duration of expiration is usually seen in COPD and in emphysema (see above for abnormalities in rate and rhythm of breathing)

There are basically three types of adventitious breath sounds:

Discontinuous: or coarse and fine crackles that indicate the presence of fluid in the lung spaces

Continuous: of which there are high- and low-pitched wheezes, which indicate narrowing or partial obstruction of the airways from inflammation, mucus, edema, foreign body, or mass

Rubs: a grating sound heard both on inspiration and expiration that is

caused by the
rubbing together
of inflamed
pleural surfaces
(see Fig. 14–16)

Clinical Notes (see Fig. 14–17)

Sudden onset of chest pain and shortness of breath must be evaluated and ruled out for pain of cardiac origin and pulmonary embolus. These patients will need to have an ECG evaluated as well as cardiac enzymes and arterial blood gas determinations. Depending on these results, further work-up may be warranted. Remember, when in doubt, it is always safest to perform the above minimal work-up rather than miss a potentially life-threatening diagnosis.

Geriatric Considerations

Normal Findings

Chest	Less mobile because of calcification of costal cartilages
	Increased anterior-posterior (AP) diameter
	Accentuation of dorsal spine, producing kyphosis
Lungs	Hyperresonance of thorax on percussion

Clinical Notes

An altered immune system, a slowed cough response, normal aging changes, and continued exposure to polluted air make the older adult more susceptible to colds, respiratory infections, and postoperative pulmonary complications. Be alert for early signs of respiratory disorders. Provide rest times between deep breaths on auscultation to prevent dizziness and/or fainting.

Pediatric Considerations

History

Mechanical ventilation as an infant?
Meconium ileus?
Has child been immunized; are immunizations up to date?

Do parents smoke?

Substance abuse: sniffing drugs (glue, cocaine, heroin)?

When the chief complaint is coughing, is the onset during the night, awaking the child from sleep, and/or with activity?

Physical Examination

PROCEDURE. Place the stethoscope on the cheek and compare to breath sounds heard through the chest wall. This helps to differentiate referred upper airway sounds from true adventitious sounds.

Rhonchi may be heard at the oral airway; rales will *not* be heard.

Normal Findings	Common Variations	Abnormalities
Newborn		
Thin chest wall	Mouth breathing	Apnea (<20 breaths per second)
Cartilaginous rib cage	Shallow breaths	Grunting
	Pectus excavatum	
	Pectus carinatum	
Infant and Child		
AP diameter = transverse diameter		Wheezing of bronchiolitis in infant, asthma in child
Xiphoid process protrudes anteriorly		Epiglottitis: upright posture, drooling, and air hunger
Expirations > inspirations		
Diaphragmatic breathing		
Paradoxical breathing		
Breath sounds louder and harsher than those of adults		
Hyperresonance throughout		
Diminished breath sounds are the equivalent of dullness in the adult		

Adolescent   Barrel chest

Clubbing

Clinical Notes

Cough from URI persists throughout the day and may get worse upon lying flat; cough from reactive airway and/or asthma typically gets worse in the early hours of the morning and with exercise/activity.

Intensity and type of airway retractions helps localize airway obstruction:

Upper airway obstruction: Supra/substernal retractions

Lower airway obstruction: Intercostal retractions predominate

Decreasing "noisy" breath sounds in a child with croup may mean *complete* airway obstruction rather than an improvement in condition.

15

Assessment of the Heart

HISTORY AND CURRENT STATUS QUESTIONS

Personal history	Congenital defect, enlarged heart, arrhythmias, murmur, stenosis or insufficiency of valves, septal defects, coronary artery disease (CAD), congestive heart failure (CHF), angina, or myocardial infarction (MI)
	Hypertension (HTN), diabetes (DM), hypercholesterolemia, a history of stroke (cerebral vascular accident [CVA])
Family history	Family members with any of the above-described illnesses (note: relation to the patient, specific problem, age of onset, age of death, disease/cause of relative's death)
Risk factors?	Congenital heart disease; rheumatic fever; thyroid disease; HTN; DM; obesity; tobacco use; hypercholesterolemia; excessive caffeine, alcohol; or drug abuse
Chest pain?	Often patients are unable to describe the sensation they feel as "pain"; evaluate all complaints of pain with regard to the following (see Fig. 15–2):

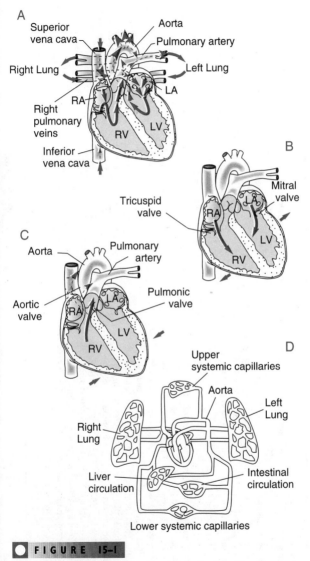

The cardiac cycle. *A*, Cardiac circulation. *B*, Diastole. *C*, Systole. *D*, Systemic circulation.

Provocative or Palliative	Quality or Quantity	Region or Radiation	Severity Scale	Timing
What causes the symptom? What makes it better or worse?	**How does the symptom feel, look, or sound? How much of it are you experiencing now?**	**Where is the symptom located? Does it spread?**	**How does the symptom rate on a severity scale of 1 to 10, with 10 being the most extreme?**	**When did the symptom begin? How often does it occur? Is it sudden or gradual?**
• First occurrence. What were you doing when you first experienced or noticed the symptom? What seems to trigger it: stress? position? certain activities? arguments? (For a physical symptom such as a discharge: What seems to cause it or make it worse? For a psychological symptom: Does the depression occur	• Quality. How would you describe the symptom—how it feels, looks, or sounds? • Quantity. How much are you experiencing now? Is it so much that it prevents you from performing any activities? Is it more or less than you experienced at any other time?	• Region. Where does the symptom occur? • Radiation. In the case of pain, does it travel down your back or arms, up your neck, or down your legs?	• Severity. How bad is the symptom at its worst? Does it force you to lie down, sit down, or slow down? • Course. Does the symptom seem to be getting better, getting worse, or staying about the same?	• Onset. On what date did the symptom first occur? What time did it begin? • Type of onset. How did the symptom start: suddenly? gradually? • Frequency. How often do you experience the symptom: hourly? daily? weekly? monthly? When do you usually experience it: during the day? at night? in the early

● **F I G U R E   15–2**

Provocative or Palliative	Quality or Quantity	Region or Radiation	Severity Scale	Timing
when you feel rejected?) What relieves the symptom: changing diet? changing position? taking medication? being active? • Aggravation. What makes the symptom worse?				morning? Does it awaken you? Does it occur before, during, or after meals? Does it occur seasonally? • Duration. How long does an episode of the symptom last?

From Morton PG. Health Assessment in Nursing. 2nd ed. Philadelphia: FA Davis, 1993.

FIGURE 15–2 *Continued*

System of evaluation of symptoms: The PQRST mnemonic.

Provocative factors: *What provoked the pain?*

Exertion, rest, eating, position changes, emotions, weather changes, etc.; type and amount of activity; change in the amount of activity required to provoke the pain over time

Palliative factors: *What can the patient do to improve or alleviate the "pain"?*

Rest, nitroglycerin, position change, warmth, stress reduction

Quality: Ask the patient to describe the pain.

Patients are often unwilling to call chest pain that is cardiac in origin "pain"; they may describe discomfort, chest pressure, tightness, viselike, crushing, something heavy sitting on their chest, or make the universal sign of a clenched fist.

Region: *Where is the pain located?*

Local or diffuse; radiates to the neck, jaw, back, shoulders, or down the arms

Severity: *Is the pain mild, moderate, or severe?*

Ask the patient to rate the pain on a scale of 1 to 10 (where 10 is the most severe)

Timing: *When did the pain start?*

Occurs at a particular time of day?

Rhythm irregularities?	Palpitations, skipped beats, racing of the heart: when, how often; associated symptoms (shortness of breath, chest pain, or diaphoresis)

Shortness of breath?	Unexpectedly; constant or intermittent; at rest or with exertion
	What type and how much activity provokes it; has this amount changed over time At night, Awakens patient from sleep; need for extra pillows; associated with cough, fever, chest pain, or diaphoresis
Cyanosis?	Blue lips or nailbeds, ashen color of skin
Cough?	Hacking, constant, intermittent, or rare; Time of day (e.g., early morning); chest pain; productive or nonproductive: color and consistency of the sputum (thick, thin, clear, yellow, green, malodorous, blood tinged); provoked by activity, position changes, weather; alleviating factors (e.g., rest, medications)
Fatigue?	Keep up with friends and colleagues; sudden or gradual onset; related to time of day
Edema?	Where and when: lower legs, ankles; at night, in the morning; pitting or nonpitting; unilateral or bilateral; any associated pain
Nocturia?	Waking at night with the urgent need to urinate
Occupational risks?	Stressful occupation; exposed to smoke, pollution, toxins, vapors, fumes, strenuous exercise
Medications?	Cardiovascular medications: type, dosage, how long; side effects; any recent changes in medications or dosages
Past work-up?	Past cardiovascular tests or surgery: chest x-ray, ECG, echocardiogram, exer-

cise stress test, Holter monitor, cardiac catheterization, angioplasty, valvuloplasty, valve replacements, or bypass

Results; complications

PHYSICAL EXAMINATION

Equipment

Stethoscope
Tape measure

Procedures, Techniques, and Findings

Procedure	*Technique*
1. Prepare the patient for the exam.	Ask the patient to undress to the waist. Be sure there is adequate lighting. The patient may be examined sitting up, or supine.
2. Inspect and palpate the anterior chest, including all six anatomical landmarks: Aortic area (right 2nd intercostal space, ICS) Pulmonic area (left 2nd ICS) Erb's point (left 3rd ICS) Tricuspid (left 5th ICS at sternum) Apical (left 5th ICS at midclavicular line, MCL) Epigastric (just below the tip of the sternum, Fig 15–3).	Inspect the undressed patient from the side and at an angle to take full advantage of lighting. Palpate the chest and all anatomical landmarks using the ball of the hand and posterior side of the proximal finger joints placed lightly on the chest surface in each area. Time the occurrence of any perceived pulsations, heaves, or thrills, with systole and diastole by simultaneously auscultating the heart or palpating the carotid artery. Heaves are forceful pulsations that bound against the hand; thrills are vibrations.

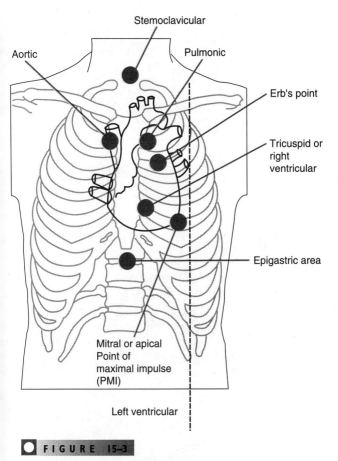

Stemoclavicular

Aortic

Pulmonic

Erb's point

Tricuspid or right ventricular

Epigastric area

Mitral or apical
Point of maximal impulse (PMI)

Left ventricular

● FIGURE 15–3

Palpation of the six anatomical landmarks.

3. Palpate the apical impulse; this is usually the point of maximum impulse (PMI) (Fig. 15–4).

Palpate the apical area (the left 5th ICS at the MCL). You should feel a tapping sensation occurring in an area that is 1 to 2 cm in diameter and confined to one intercostal space.

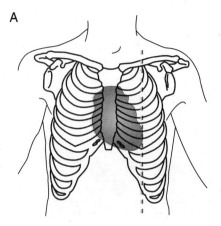

A

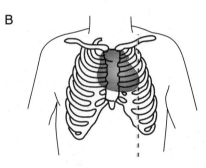

B

C

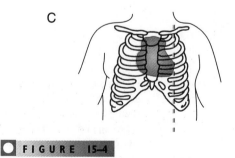

FIGURE 15-4

Location of the apex of the heart. *A*, Adult. *B*, Child. *C*, Infant.

4. Palpate the carotid pulse.

Ask the patient to turn his head away from the side chosen for palpation. Observe the neck for pulsations. Place the tips of two fingers held together (usually the index and second finger) lightly over the pulsations. Auscultate the heart simultaneously and determine whether the carotid pulse is regular and synchronous to the first heart sound (S1).

5. Percuss out the cardiac border and assess the size of the heart.

Rarely is this technique ever employed in practice because chest x-rays now provide a much more reliable assessment of cardiac size and contour; however, in areas where chest x-rays are not readily available this is a useful technique to know.

Using the percussion technique described in Chapter 14, Assessment of the Chest and Lungs, percuss out the borders of cardiac dullness and assess the size of the heart. The heart tissue will be dull to percussion amid surrounding resonant lung tissue. The left border of cardiac dullness is usually at the 5th ICS at the MCL and 2nd ICS at the sternum. The right border of cardiac dullness is usually at the sternum.

6. Auscultate the heart for rate and rhythm (Fig. 15-5).

Using the diaphragm of the stethoscope, auscultate in the apical area of the heart (left 5th ICS at MCL) for the rate and rhythm; counting the first (S1) and second (S2) heart sounds, "lub-dub," in combination as one "beat," assess the heart rate by counting the number of beats there are in a full minute.

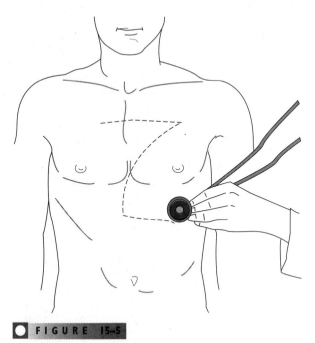

FIGURE 15-5

Auscultation of the heart for rate and rhythm.

Assess the cardiac rhythm. Listen to several full cycles, paying particular attention to the lengths of the systolic pauses between S1 and S2, and the longer diastolic pauses between S2 and S1. Both the length of systolic and diastolic pauses should be consistent in all cycles. Any variation in length of systolic or diastolic pauses, abnormally long pauses, or sudden increase in heart rate over a number of cycles constitutes an irregular rhythm (Fig. 15–6).

7. Compare the apical and radial pulse if the rhythm of the heart is found to be irregular.

Compare the apical and radial pulse by simultaneously auscultating the heart rate in the apical area while taking the patient's radial pulse. Compare the rates (beats per full minute) between the apical and radial pulse. If there is a deficit, it is usually the radial pulse that has the lower rate.

8. Auscultate the heart in each of the six anatomical landmarks; at each site listen for:

   Rate and rhythm

   S1 and S2

   Systole and diastole

   Extra heart sounds

   Murmurs

Auscultate the heart over each of the six anatomical landmarks, first with the diaphragm of the stethoscope, and then with the bell (see Fig. 15–3). Apply firm pressure when using the diaphragm, and light pressure when using the bell. It is no longer advised to limit auscultation to the landmarks alone because the sounds produced by the

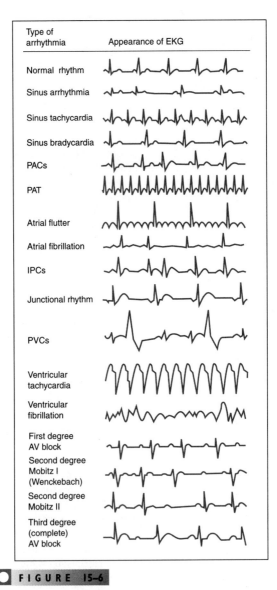

Type of arrhythmia	Appearance of EKG
Normal rhythm	
Sinus arrhythmia	
Sinus tachycardia	
Sinus bradycardia	
PACs	
PAT	
Atrial flutter	
Atrial fibrillation	
IPCs	
Junctional rhythm	
PVCs	
Ventricular tachycardia	
Ventricular fibrillation	
First degree AV block	
Second degree Mobitz I (Wenckebach)	
Second degree Mobitz II	
Third degree (complete) AV block	

FIGURE 15-6

Assessment of cardiac rhythm and irregularities.

closing of heart valves may often be heard all over the precordium; instead, edge your stethoscope across the base of the heart and down to the apex in a "Z-like" path that will include the anatomical landmarks, while at the same time covering more surface area of the heart. Listen to each heart sound carefully (Fig. 15–5).

9. Identify and carefully auscultate the first (S1) and second (S2) heart sound.

The first heart sound (S1) or "lub" is followed by the shorter pause or systole. It occurs at the same time as the carotid pulse. It is heard best at the apex of the heart and is louder than the second heart sound (S2) or "dub" at the apical and tricuspid area and at Erb's point. It is softer than S2 at the pulmonic and aortic areas.

S2 or "dub" is followed by the longer pause or diastole. It is heard best in the aortic area. It is louder than S1 at the aortic and pulmonic areas and softer than S1 in the apical and tricuspid areas and at Erb's point.

Once you have identified S1 and S2, listen to them carefully and separately. Note whether the heart sounds are normal, accentuated (loud), or split (Fig. 15–7).

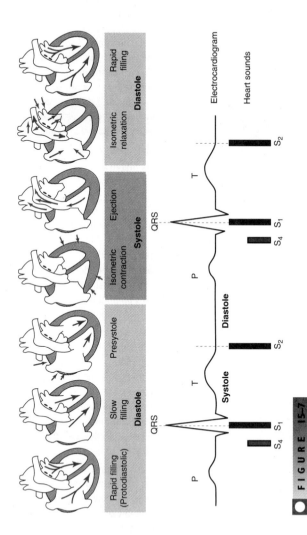

FIGURE 15-7

Normal heart sounds.

10. Identify and auscultate systole and diastole.

Systole is the shorter pause between S1 and S2.

Diastole is the longer pause between S2 and S1.

Usually systole and diastole are silent (see Fig. 15–7).

11. Auscultate for extra heart sounds. Note whether there are split sounds, third (S3), or fourth (S4), heart sounds, or clicks audible.

Usually both the systolic and diastolic pauses are silent. Auscultate carefully over a number of full cycles to determine whether any extra heart sounds are occurring. You may hear a split S1 or S2, systolic clicks, prosthetic valve sounds, or an S3 or S4 (the most common sounds occurring in diastole). An S3 follows the S2 and an S4 precedes the S1. Evaluate each extra sound for location, timing, and characteristics. Be specific with descriptions of timing. State whether the sound occurs in early, mid, or late systole or diastole (see Fig. 15–8).

12. Auscultate for heart murmurs; grade the intensity of each murmur and evaluate for pattern, quality, location, radiation, and posture.

Murmurs occur when there is turbulent blood flow in the heart or great vessels. They are heard as a swooshing or blowing sound when auscultated. Evaluate all murmurs for intensity, pattern, quality, location, radiation, and posture.

Intensity: The intensity of a murmur may be high, medium, or low, depending on the pressure and rate of

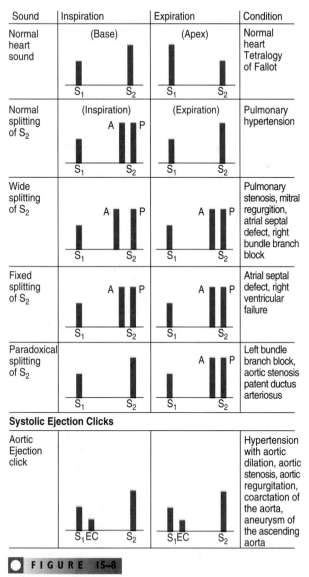

Sound	Inspiration	Expiration	Condition
Normal heart sound	(Base) S_1 S_2	(Apex) S_1 S_2	Normal heart Tetralogy of Fallot
Normal splitting of S_2	(Inspiration) A P S_1 S_2	(Expiration) S_1 S_2	Pulmonary hypertension
Wide splitting of S_2	A P S_1 S_2	A P S_1 S_2	Pulmonary stenosis, mitral regurgitation, atrial septal defect, right bundle branch block
Fixed splitting of S_2	A P S_1 S_2	A P S_1 S_2	Atrial septal defect, right ventricular failure
Paradoxical splitting of S_2	S_1 S_2	A P S_1 S_2	Left bundle branch block, aortic stenosis patent ductus arteriosus

Systolic Ejection Clicks

Aortic Ejection click	S_1EC S_2	S_1EC S_2	Hypertension with aortic dilation, aortic stenosis, aortic regurgitation, coarctation of the aorta, aneurysm of the ascending aorta

● **FIGURE 15–8**

Abnormal heart sounds.

Illustration continued on following page

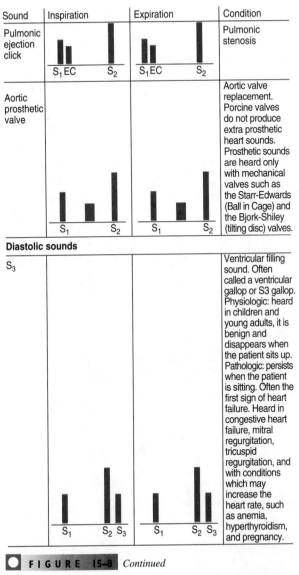

Sound	Inspiration	Expiration	Condition
Pulmonic ejection click	S_1 EC S_2	S_1 EC S_2	Pulmonic stenosis
Aortic prosthetic valve	S_1 S_2	S_1 S_2	Aortic valve replacement. Porcine valves do not produce extra prosthetic heart sounds. Prosthetic sounds are heard only with mechanical valves such as the Starr-Edwards (Ball in Cage) and the Bjork-Shiley (tilting disc) valves.

Diastolic sounds

| S_3 | S_1 S_2 S_3 | S_1 S_2 S_3 | Ventricular filling sound. Often called a ventricular gallop or S3 gallop. Physiologic: heard in children and young adults, it is benign and disappears when the patient sits up. Pathologic: persists when the patient is sitting. Often the first sign of heart failure. Heard in congestive heart failure, mitral regurgitation, tricuspid regurgitation, and with conditions which may increase the heart rate, such as anemia, hyperthyroidism, and pregnancy. |

⬤ **FIGURE 15-8** *Continued*

Illustration continued on following page

Sound	Inspiration	Expiration	Condition
S_4	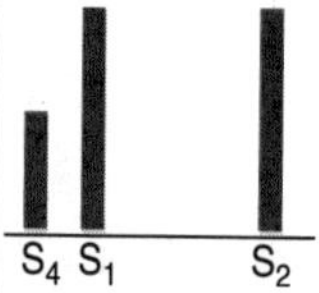 S_4 S_1 S_2	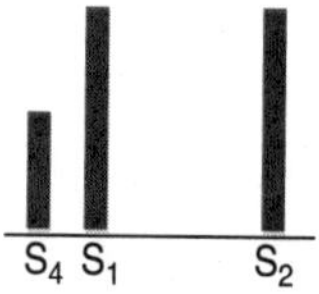 S_4 S_1 S_2	Ventricular filling sound. Often called an atrial gallop or S4 gallop. May be Physiologic: Benign. Occuring in patients over 40 years old without cardiac disease. Pathologic: Occurs with decreases compliance of the ventricle, as in cardiomyopathy, coronary artery disease, aortic stenosis, systemic hypertension, pulmonary stenosis, or pulmonary hypertension.
Opening snap of mitral valve prolapse	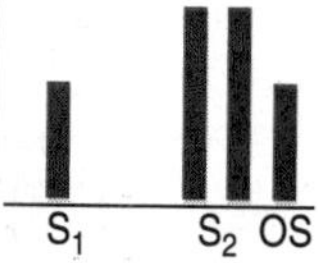 S_1 S_2 OS	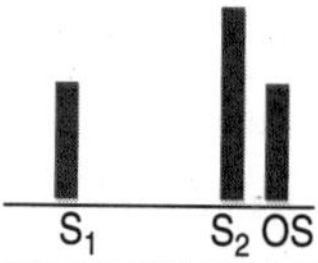 S_1 S_2 OS	Mitral valve prolapse
Prosthetic mitral valve	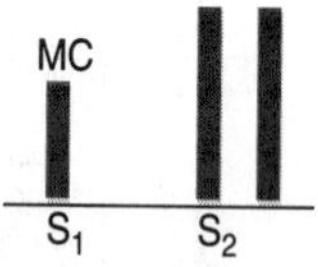 MC S_1 S_2	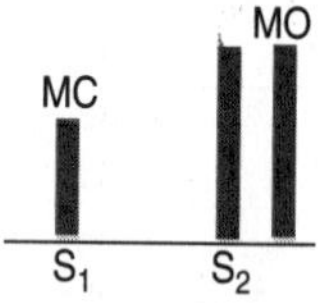 MC S_1 S_2 MO	Mitral valve replacement

FIGURE 15-8 *Continued*

blood flow. To more accurately describe the intensity, murmurs are generally graded according to the rating scale below (i.e., a moderately loud murmur would be rated III/VI):

I: Barely audible

II: Audible but faint

III: Moderately loud

IV: Loud and associated with a thrill

V: Loud and heard with the corner of the stethoscope lifted off the chest wall

VI: Loudest and heard easily without a stethoscope, or with a stethoscope held 1 inch above the chest wall

They may also vary in their intensity. They may grow louder in intensity (crescendo), taper off in intensity (decrescendo), or increase in intensity to an apex and then taper off all within one systolic or diastolic pause (crescendo–decrescendo or diamond shaped.)

Pattern: They may be pansystolic or holosystolic (or pandiastolic or holodiastolic) and occur throughout the entire length of the systolic (or diastolic) pause, or in the early, mid, or late part of systole (or diastole). (Fig 15–9).

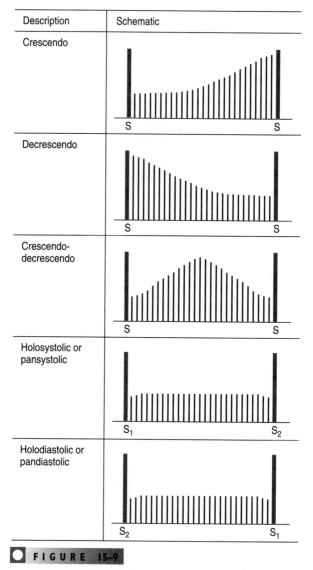

Description	Schematic
Crescendo	S S
Decrescendo	S S
Crescendo-decrescendo	S S
Holosystolic or pansystolic	S_1 S_2
Holodiastolic or pandiastolic	S_2 S_1

● FIGURE 15-9

Auscultation for heart murmur intensity and pattern.

	Normal Findings	**Abnormal Findings**
Inspection and palpation of the anterior chest	✓ No lesions, masses, or abnormalities; there should be a palpable pulsation, felt as a light tapping sensation, in the apical landmark at the left 5th ICS at the MCL	Any lesions, masses, or abnormalities of the chest; any palpable heaves (strong thrusting sensations) or thrills (vibratory sensations) anywhere in the precordium; any pulsations palpable in any location other than the apical landmark
Apical impulse	The apical impulse is usually the PMI; it is confined to one ICS, in an area 1 to 2 cm in diameter	Displacement of the apical impulse or an impulse felt in an area which is larger than 2 cm in diameter; may be displaced secondary to abnormal curvatures of the spine, cardiomegaly, emphysema, obesity, increased musculature, or enlarged breasts; may be faint or barely perceivable secondary to pericardial effusions, pulmonary effusions, tumors, or any condition that may increase tissue mass or fluid be-

		tween the heart and the chest wall
Carotid pulse	Regular bounding rhythm that is synchronous to S1	Irregular rhythm: carotid pulse not synchronous to S1
		Carotid bruit: represents turbulence in the artery from atherosclerotic plaque or thrombosis
		Murmur: represents a cardiac disorder; may be transmitted to the carotid artery
Cardiac size	Chest x-ray provides the most accurate assessment of cardiac size; if the percussion technique is used, the left border of cardiac dullness is usually at the 5th ICS at the MCL; the right side is on the sternal border (see Fig. 15–4)	Cardiomegaly, left ventricular hypertrophy, pericardial effusion, or mass, may account for increased cardiac size; a small number of patients may have congenital anomalies such as dextrocardia and situs inversus, which will cause markedly abnormal findings when the borders of cardiac dullness are percussed
Heart rate and rhythm	The average heart rate for adults is between 60 and 100 beats/minute; The average heart	Sinus bradycardia: regular rhythm, with a decreased rate (<60 beats/ minute); this may

rate for children varies depending on the age; The rhythm should be regular, with systolic and diastolic pauses consistent in length

Sinus bradycardia: may be normal in well-conditioned athletes

Sinus tachycardia: may occur normally after exercise

Sinus dysrhythmia: the pulse rate changes with respirations, increasing at the peak of inspiration and decreasing with expiration; occurs often in children and young adults as a normal variant

be normal in well-conditioned athletes, however is abnormal when associated with hypothermia, hypothyroidism, drug overdoses (narcotics, digoxin)

Sinus tachycardia: regular rhythm with an increased heart rate (>100 beats/minute); this may be normal with increased exercise, however is abnormal in association with increased caffeine, stimulant overdoses, fever, pain, hyperthyroidism, anxiety, shock, and heart disease

Ventricular premature contractions (PVCs): These result in irregular heart rhythms; perceived as heart beats that occur out of sequence or rhythm; may occur singularly or in "couplets" or pairs, may be infrequent or frequent; caused

		by abnormal electrical conduction through the ventricular tissue and may indicate or be a precursor to a serious arrhythmia (see Fig. 15–6)
Comparison of apical and radial pulse	Usually the apical and radial pulse will be equivalent in rate and rhythm	If a pulse deficit occurs, it is usually the radial pulse which turns out to be less than the apical pulse. Any pulse deficit should be reported to a physician for further evaluation
First heart sound (S1) (see Fig. 15–8)	S1 is heard at the start of the shorter systolic pause; louder than S2 in the apical and tricuspid area and at Erb's point; softer than S2 in the pulmonic and aortic areas; normally synchronous to the carotid pulse; may be normally split (though this is rare) when the closing of the mitral and tricuspid valves are not synchronous	Loud S1: may be heard in hyperkinetic states and conditions that increase blood velocity such as exercise, fever, anemia, hyperthyroid, 1st degree heart block, mitral insufficiency, and severe hypertension Faint S1: may be heard in severe hypertension, 1st degree heart block, and mitral insufficiency, or any con-

| Second heart sound (S2) (see Fig. 15–8) | S2 is heard at the start of the longer diastolic pause; louder than S1 in the pulmonic and aortic areas and is softer than S1 in the apical and tricuspid areas and at Erb's point; may be normally split at the end of inspiration and return to synchronous closure (a single S2 sound) on expiration in some individuals | dition that may increase the amount of tissue or fluid between the heart and the chest wall |

Varying intensity of S1: may be heard in atrial fibrillation or complete heart block with a changing systolic pause (PR interval)

Fixed split S2: an S2 with a fixed split, or a split that is unaffected by respirations; may occur with atrial septal defects or right ventricular failure

Paradoxically split S2: a paradoxical split S2 will occur with expiration and disappear on inspiration; may occur with aortic stenosis, patent ductus arteriosus, or left bundle branch block

Faint S2: may occur with any condition that increases the amount of tissue or fluid between the heart

		and the chest wall (tumor, effusion)
Systole (see Fig. 15–8)	The systolic pause is the shorter pause occurring between S1 and S2; usually silent, without extra sounds or murmurs	Early systolic sounds: ejection clicks may occur with aortic prosthetic valves or with aortic or pulmonic stenosis; the aortic ejection click is best heard at the apex and its intensity does not change with respiration; the pulmonic ejection click is best heard in the second left interspace and grows softer with inspiration
		Midsystolic sounds: midsystolic ejection clicks occur with mitral valve prolapse
Diastole (see Fig. 15–8)	The diastolic pause is the longer pause occurring after S2 and before the next S1	Early diastolic sounds: Opening snap: the opening snap of mitral stenosis is a sharp, high-pitched snapping sound that occurs after S2 and is heard best in the third or fourth left ICS

Opening click: an opening click heard just after S2; may represent the opening sound of a ball-in-cage mitral valve prosthesis

Summation sound (S3 + S4): occurs with cardiac stress and increased heart rates; the pathologic S3 and S4 merge into one longer louder sound that is often louder than either S1 or S2

Middiastolic sounds: S3 is a ventricular filling sound that is a dull, soft, low sound; occurs after S2 but later than an opening snap; often confused with a split S2, however, it is lower pitched than the S2, does not vary with respirations, and, unlike the S2 (which is heard best at the base of the heart), is heard best with the bell of the stethoscope at the apex or left lower sternal border; may be normal or physiologic in children and young adults— if so it will usually disappear when the patient is sitting up, whereas the abnormal S3 or pathologic S3 (called the ventricular gallop) will not disappear with the patient sitting up

Late diastolic sounds: S4 is a very soft low sound heard just before S1; ventricular filling sound heard best with the bell of the stethoscope with the patient in the left lateral recumbent position; a physiologic S4 may occur in adults over age 40 with no evidence of cardiovascular disease; a pathologic S4, or atrial gallop, occurs with conditions that decrease compliance of the ventricle such as coronary artery disease, cardiomyopathy, systolic overload, and systemic HTN

Pacemaker-induced sound: rarely heard today because of improved pacemaker design; in the past heard as high-pitched clicks representing muscle contractions induced by the pacemakers

Pericardial friction rub: a high-pitched scratchy sound resembling sandpaper; occurs with pericarditis (inflammation of the pericardium); best heard with the diaphragm and with the patient sitting up and leaning forward and holding breath

Systolic murmurs (Fig. 15–10)

Normally none heard

Patent ductus arteriosus (PDA): produces a continuous systolic murmur often called a machinery murmur

Text continued on page 306

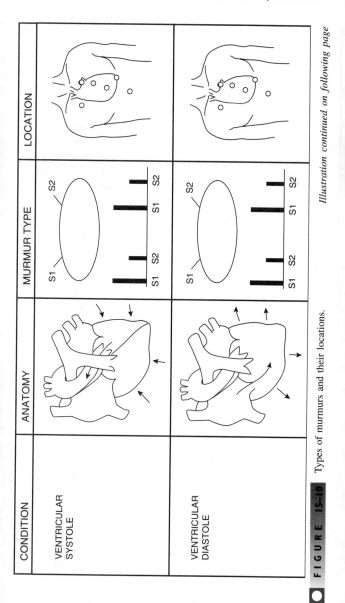

CONDITION	ANATOMY	MURMUR TYPE	LOCATION
VENTRICULAR SYSTOLE		S1 — S2 S1 — S2	
VENTRICULAR DIASTOLE		S1 — S2 S1 — S2	

Illustration continued on following page

FIGURE 15–10 Types of murmurs and their locations.

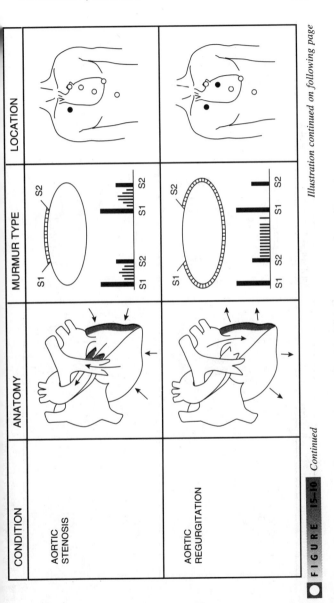

CONDITION	ANATOMY	MURMUR TYPE	LOCATION
AORTIC STENOSIS			
AORTIC REGURGITATION			

Illustration continued on following page

FIGURE 15–10 *Continued*

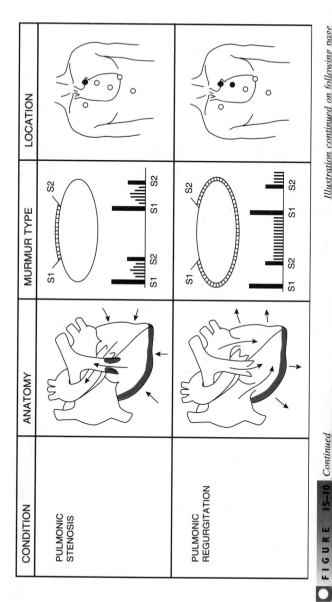

CONDITION	ANATOMY	MURMUR TYPE	LOCATION
PULMONIC STENOSIS		S1 S2 / S1 S2	
PULMONIC REGURGITATION		S1 S2 / S1 S2	

FIGURE 15–10 Continued

Illustration continued on following page

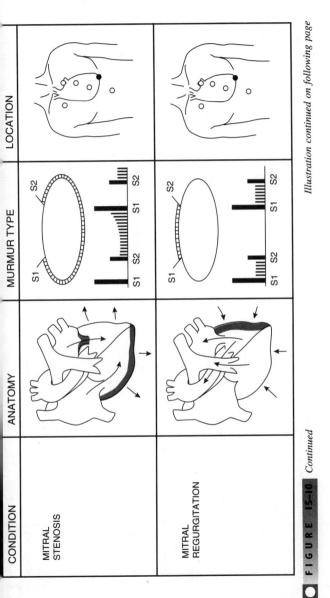

Illustration continued on following page

FIGURE 15-10 *Continued*

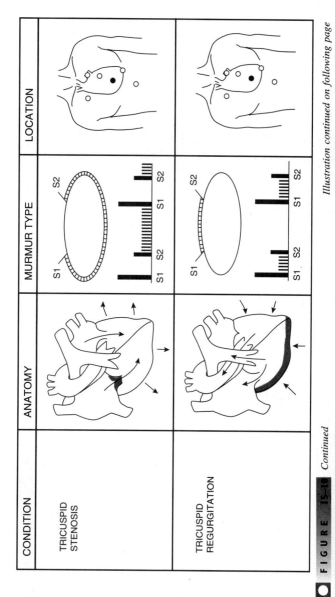

CONDITION	ANATOMY	MURMUR TYPE	LOCATION
TRICUSPID STENOSIS			
TRICUSPID REGURGITATION			

Illustration continued on following page

FIGURE 15–10 Continued

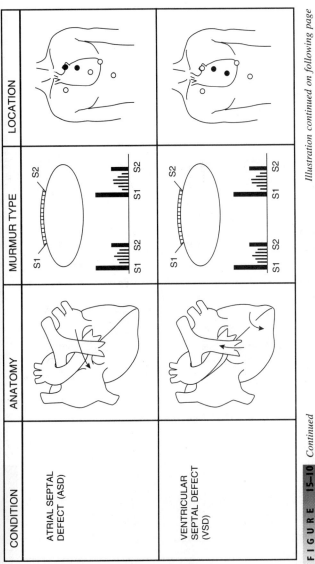

CONDITION	ANATOMY	MURMUR TYPE	LOCATION
ATRIAL SEPTAL DEFECT (ASD)			
VENTRICULAR SEPTAL DEFECT (VSD)			

Illustration continued on following page

FIGURE 15-10 *Continued*

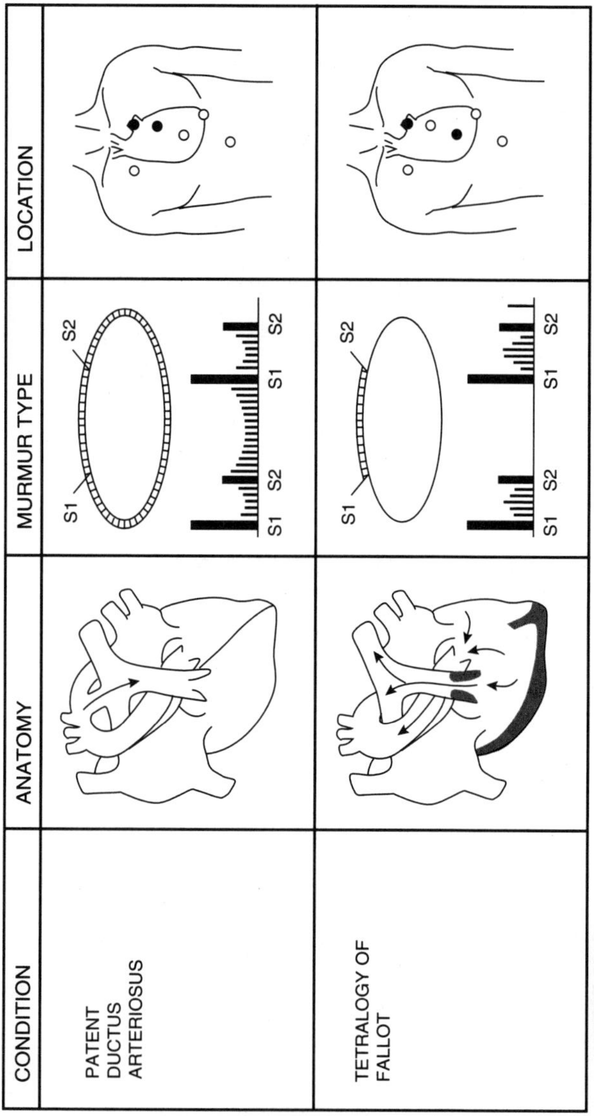

CONDITION
ANATOMY
MURMUR TYPE
LOCATION
PATENT DUCTUS ARTERIOSUS
S1
S2
S1 S2 S1 S2
TETRALOGY OF FALLOT
S1
S2
S1 S2 S1 S2

FIGURE 15-10 *Continued*

Illustration continued on following page

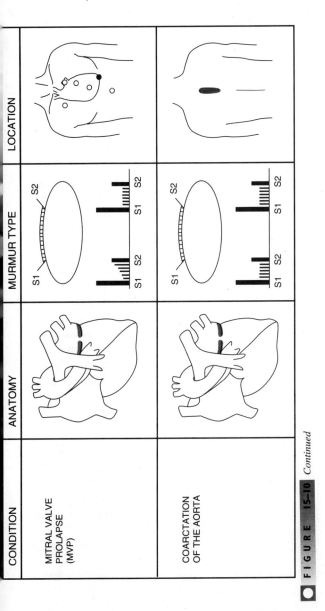

CONDITION	ANATOMY	MURMUR TYPE	LOCATION
MITRAL VALVE PROLAPSE (MVP)		S1 S2 / S1 S2 / S1 S2	
COARCTATION OF THE AORTA		S1 S2 / S1 S2 / S1 S2	

FIGURE 15-10 *Continued*

Atrial septal defect (ASD): produces a medium-pitched, systolic ejection murmur, best heard at the second left ICS

Ventricular septal defect (VSD): produces a loud, harsh, holosystolic murmur best heard at the left lower sternal border; in very large VSDs a soft diastolic murmur will often also be audible at the apex

Tetralogy of Fallot: produces a loud, crescendo–decrescendo, systolic murmur

Aortic stenosis: produces a loud midsystolic crescendo–decrescendo murmur, heard best at the second right ICS, which radiates to the side of the neck, left sternal border, or apex

Pulmonic stenosis: produces a medium-pitch

coarse, crescendo–decrescendo murmur, best heard at the second left ICS, which often radiates to the left and the neck

Mitral regurgitation: produces a pansystolic loud, blowing, murmur, best heard at the apex, which radiates to the left axilla

Tricuspid regurgitation: produces a soft blowing, pansystolic murmur, best heard at the left lower sternal border, which increases with inspiration

Diastolic murmurs
(see Fig. 15–10)

Mitral stenosis: produces a low-pitched, rumbling, diastolic murmur, best heard at the apex with the patient in the left lateral recumbent position

Tricuspid stenosis: produces a rumbling, diastolic murmur, best heard at the left lower sternal border, which

grows louder with
inspiration

Aortic or pulmonic
regurgitation: pro-
duces a soft, high-
pitched, blowing,
diastolic, decre-
scendo murmur,
best heard at the
third left ICS at
the base

Clinical Notes

An ECG should be performed and evaluated to complete
a thorough cardiac examination and to definitively identify
arrythmias. Furthermore, an absolute diagnosis should never be
made on the basis of extra heart sounds and murmurs alone. An
echocardiogram or cardiac catheterization may be useful in
obtaining definitive diagnoses of the causes of extra heart
sounds and murmurs.

Geriatric Considerations

	Normal Findings
Rate	Longer to speed up and return to baseline in response to stress or exercise
Sound	Systolic murmurs often present because of a thickening of valves
PMI	May be displaced downward because of kyphosis

Clinical Note

Heart sounds may sound distant because of structural changes
in the chest wall. To enhance the intensity of heart sounds, assist
and support the patient to sit up and lean forward.

Pediatric Considerations

History

Maternal therapeutic drugs during pregnancy?
Maternal substance abuse during pregnancy?
Poor feeding?
General activity level, exercise tolerance?
Squatting during play?
Circumoral cyanosis, central cyanosis versus peripheral cyanosis?
Irritability?

Physical Examination

EQUIPMENT.

Newborn, infant, child, adult blood pressure cuffs
Doppler sphygmomanometer

PROCEDURE.

Blood pressure must be taken on all four extremities after birth and during infancy.
Pinch nose to obliterate breath sounds for 2 seconds while evaluating the heart sounds of newborn.

Normal Findings	Common Variations	Abnormal Findings
Newborn, Infant, and Child		
Heart sounds: louder, high pitched, shorter duration		Unequal pulses in upper and lower extremities
		Unequal BPs in upper and lower extremities; between arms
Sinus arrhythmia	PVCs	Gallop rhythm
	Splitting of S2	
Capillary refill: 1 to 2 seconds		Weak suck
		Flaccid posturing

		Exercise intolerance
		Abdominal organomegaly
	Peripheral cyanosis	Circumoral or central cyanosis
		Tachypnea
		Tachycardia
		Failure to thrive

Child

PMI visible, palpated at 4th ICS until 7 years old	S1 > S2 at apex

PMI:
 	
  < 4 years: left of MCL
 	
  4 to 6 years: at MCL
 	
  > 7 years: right of MCL
	Innocent murmur: heard in the absence of findings for cardiac disease; *systolic,* LSB, 2nd to 4th ICS, Gr. II; loudest in supine and does not radiate

	Venous hum: often heard over aortic or pulmonic spaces; can be obliterated by rotating the head

Clinical Notes

Contrary to adults, pulmonary and peripheral edema are such *late* signs of cardiac failure in children that they are not considered useful indicators for diagnosis. Early signs include enlarged liver, gallop rhythm, and venous engorgement. Newborn and infant breath sounds may easily be mistaken for a murmur.

16

Assessment of the Peripheral Vascular System

HISTORY AND CURRENT STATUS QUESTIONS

Personal history	Hypertension, coronary artery disease, atherosclerotic heart disease (ASHD), high cholesterol levels, diabetes, pulmonary embolus (PE), stroke or cerebral vascular accidents (CVA), phlebitis, deep vein thrombosis (DVT), aneurysm, varicosities, vasculitis, or systemic lupus erythematous (SLE); previous vascular procedures or surgery (type); anticoagulants (which ones, for what condition)
Family history	Family members with any of the conditions mentioned above (family member, relation

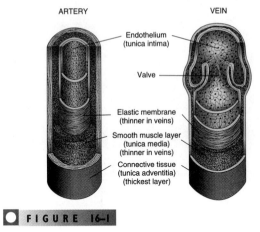

ARTERY VEIN

Endothelium (tunica intima)

Valve

Elastic membrane (thinner in veins)

Smooth muscle layer (tunica media) (thinner in veins)

Connective tissue (tunica adventitia) (thickest layer)

FIGURE 16–1

A, Arteries and veins.

Illustration continued on following page

	to the patient, condition, treatment rendered)
Cyanosis?	Blue nailbeds of the fingers and toes
Edema or swelling?	Bilateral or unilateral; pitting or nonpitting; associated pain
Paresthesias?	Numbness or tingling of any of the extremities
Pain or leg cramps?	Time of occurrence (at night while sleeping, during the day when the patient is active); pain relief measures (massage, heat, quinine); tight stockings or garter belts worn; tendency

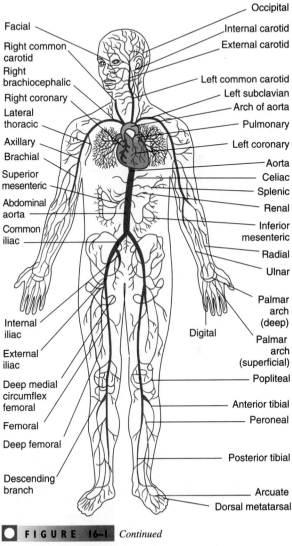

FIGURE 16-1 *Continued*

B, Systemic arterial circulation.

Illustration continued on following page

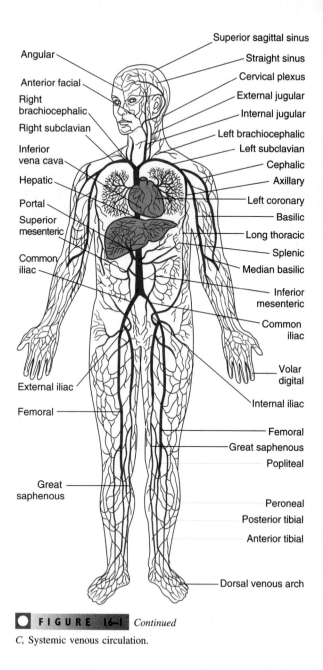

Angular
Anterior facial
Right brachiocephalic
Right subclavian
Inferior vena cava
Hepatic
Portal
Superior mesenteric
Common iliac
External iliac
Femoral
Great saphenous

Superior sagittal sinus
Straight sinus
Cervical plexus
External jugular
Internal jugular
Left brachiocephalic
Left subclavian
Cephalic
Axillary
Left coronary
Basilic
Long thoracic
Splenic
Median basilic
Inferior mesenteric
Common iliac
Volar digital
Internal iliac
Femoral
Great saphenous
Popliteal
Peroneal
Posterior tibial
Anterior tibial
Dorsal venous arch

FIGURE 16–1 *Continued*

C, Systemic venous circulation.

	to cross legs for extended periods of time
Temperature change?	Cold or heat intolerance or unusually cold fingers or toes (extremities equally affected, or noticeable difference in temperature between paired extremities)
Lesions and infections?	Prone to superficial infections, lesions, or ulcers on lower extremities (feet and ankles) that are slow to heal
Stasis dermatitis?	Progressively brownish discoloration of the skin (or rubor) caused by impaired circulation
CNS impairment?	Neurological deficits, dizziness, syncope, headaches, vision changes, change in mental status (may indicate a CVA)

PHYSICAL EXAMINATION

Equipment

Stethoscope

Sphygmomanometer

Procedures, Techniques, and Findings

Procedure	*Technique*
1. Prepare the patient for the examination.	Ask the patient to undress to underwear and sit, stand, or lie down as necessary throughout the examination of the peripheral vascular system.
2. Assess the patient's blood pressure (BP) (see Chapter 3, Fig. 3–9).	Using your stethoscope and sphygmomanometer, measure the patient's BP while the patient is relaxed and sitting and

again just after standing.
Compare BPs in each arm. Assess whether there are orthostatic changes in BP (represented by a diastolic change of >10 mmHg between sitting and standing pressures).

3. Inspect and palpate the carotid arteries.

With the patient sitting, inspect and palpate the pulsations of the carotid arteries (Fig. 16–2). Use the index and middle fingers together to gently palpate the carotid arteries on either side of the neck near the medial edge of the sternocleidomastoid muscle. Examine one artery at a time. (It may help to turn the patient's head slightly away from you for inspection, and then back toward you for palpation.) Compare and note the rate, rhythm, and strength of pulsations of

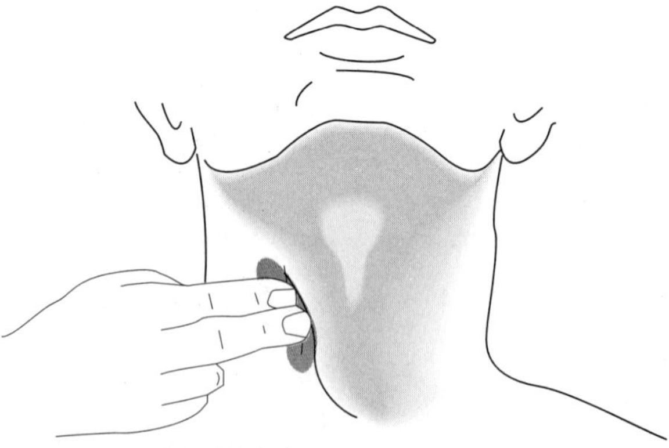

● **FIGURE 16–2**

Carotid pulse.

both carotid arteries. Note whether the rate is synchronous with the patient's heart beat and whether the rate changes with inspiration or expiration. Ask the patient to hold his/her breath, and auscultate each carotid artery for bruits using the bell of the stethoscope.

4. Assess the jugular venous pulsations.

Inspect the jugular veins with the patient sitting up at a 90 degree angle and again with the patient lying down with the head raised slightly at a 30 to 45 degree angle. Assess the level of jugular vein distension on both sides using the two-ruler method (Fig. 16–3). Note any pressures that measure > 3 cm or 1¼ inches.

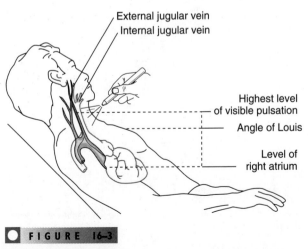

External jugular vein
Internal jugular vein

Highest level of visible pulsation

Angle of Louis

Level of right atrium

FIGURE 16–3

Inspection of the jugular vein.

5. Assess the peripheral venous circulation.

Inspect and palpate for signs of peripheral venous insufficiency (changes in the skin, changes in temperature, presence of edema, varicosities, phlebitis, and thrombosis).

Skin changes

Assess the skin, nailbeds, and extremities for signs of venous insufficiency (Fig. 16–4). Note

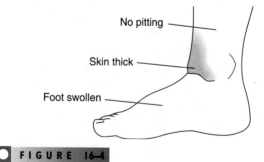

FIGURE 16–4

Inspection for edema and venous insufficiency. *A*, Orthostatic edema *B*, Lymphedema.

Illustration continued on following page

whether there is any pallor, cyanosis, stasis dermatitis, ulcers, necrosis, edema, or cellulitis.

Temperature   Note whether the patient's fingers or toes are unusually cool to the touch. Compare paired extremities, fingers, and toes and note whether temperature changes are unilateral or bilateral.

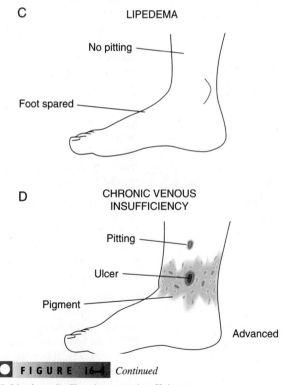

C   LIPEDEMA

No pitting

Foot spared

D   CHRONIC VENOUS
INSUFFICIENCY

Pitting

Ulcer

Pigment

Advanced

⬤ **FIGURE 16-4** *Continued*

C, Lipedema *D*, Chronic venous insufficiency.

Edema	Note whether there is any edema of the lower extremities. Assess whether it is pitting or nonpitting (Fig. 16–5). Note the extent of involvement (the edema of peripheral vascular disease is usually ascending. It may begin in the ankles and ascend up the leg, depending on the severity of vascular compromise).
Varicosities	Inspect and palpate the lower extremities for varicosities. They appear as swollen, thick, tortuous veins easily seen and palpated along the surface of the lower extremities.
Phlebitis	Inspect and palpate the superficial veins for signs of phlebitis or inflammation. Look for reddened, thickened, or tender veins. If any occur in the lower legs, palpate the calf muscles for tenderness.
Thrombosis	Perform a special maneuver to detect DVT. With the patient's knee flexed, dorsiflex the foot. In the presence of a DVT there will be characteristic calf pain ("Homan's sign").
Special maneuvers	Phlebitis: To check for the presence of phlebitis, gently squeeze the calf muscle against the tibia and note the presence of any tenderness. DVT: To check for DVT look for "Homan's sign." With the knee

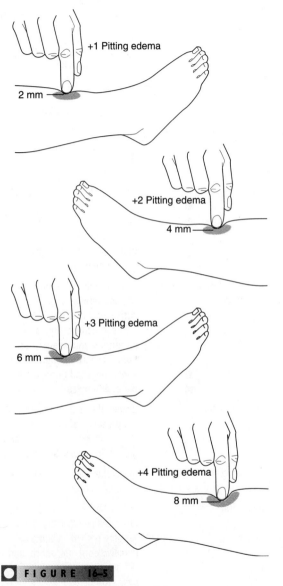

+1 Pitting edema
2 mm

+2 Pitting edema
4 mm

+3 Pitting edema
6 mm

+4 Pitting edema
8 mm

FIGURE 16-5

Inspection for pitting or nonpitting edema.

slightly flexed, dorsiflex the foot and note any occurrence of calf tenderness. The presence of calf tenderness constitutes a "positive" Homan's sign, and suggests the presence of a DVT.

Trendelenburg test: If varicosities are present, palpate the vessel with one hand while pressing down on the vessel with your second hand at a point just above the first hand. Palpate for the impulse of blood flow. Normally there should be none.

6. Assess the peripheral arterial circulation.

Inspect and palpate for signs of peripheral arterial insufficiency: changes in the skin and nails, changes in temperature, diminished sensation, presence of edema, pain, and diminished or absent peripheral pulses.

Skin and nails

Inspect the skin and nails. Note the presence of thin, shiny skin, scaly skin, decreased hair growth, or thickened nails.

Temperature

Note whether the extremities are cool to touch.

Sensation

Note whether the patient demonstrates any sensory deficits. Test the patient's ability to perceive soft, dull, sharp, and vibratory sensations with their eyes closed.

Pulses (Fig. 16–6)	Since each person's anatomy may vary slightly, pulses are primarily located by touch. Exert light pressure with your index and middle fingertips held together and palpate the arterial pulses. You may need to use deep palpation to locate the femoral artery. Compare all contralateral or paired pulses for rhythm, strength, and equality (Fig. 16–6). If the pulse is difficult to find, or not readily palpable, you may use a doppler, or ultrasound, stethoscope to auscultate for the pulse.
Radial pulse	Palpate the radial pulse along the radial groove on the palmar and radial side of the wrist (Fig. 16–7A).
Ulnar pulse	Palpate the ulnar pulse on the palmar and medial side of the wrist (Fig. 16–7B).
Brachial pulse	Palpate the brachial pulse at the antecubital fossa between the biceps and triceps muscles (Fig. 16–7C).
Femoral pulse	Palpate the femoral pulse with the patient supine just below the inguinal ligament and halfway between the symphysis pubis and the anterior superior iliac spine. You may need to use two or three fingers and deeply palpate for the femoral pulse (Fig. 16–7D).

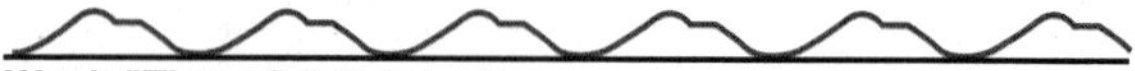

Weak "Thready" Pulse—1+
Decreased cardiac output; peripheral arterial disease;
aortic valve stenosis

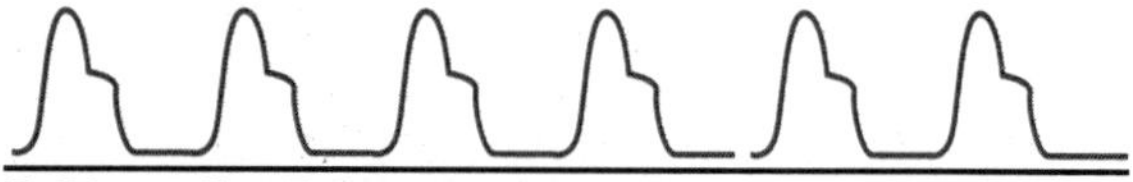

Full bounding Pulse—3+ or 4+
Hyperkinetic states (exercise, anxiety, fever), anemia,
hyperthyroidism

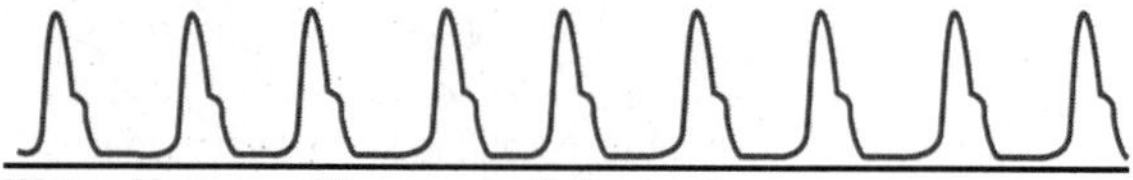

Water-Hammer (Corrigan's Pulse)—4+
Aortic valve regurgitation; patent ductus arteriosus.

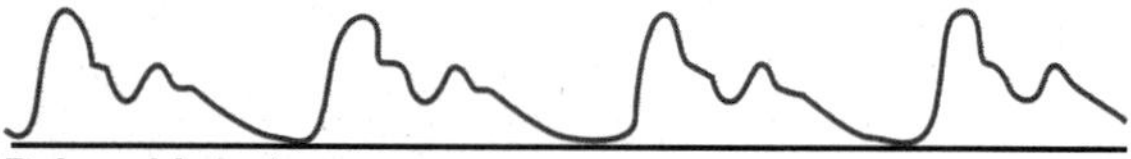

Pulsus bigeminus
Conduction disturbance, e.g., premature ventricular contraction,
premature atrial contraction.

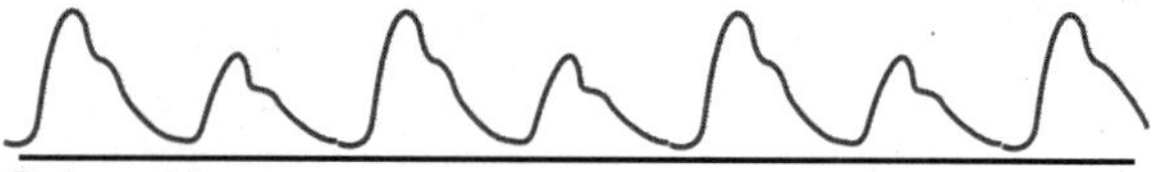

Pulsus Alternans
Left-sided congestive heart failure

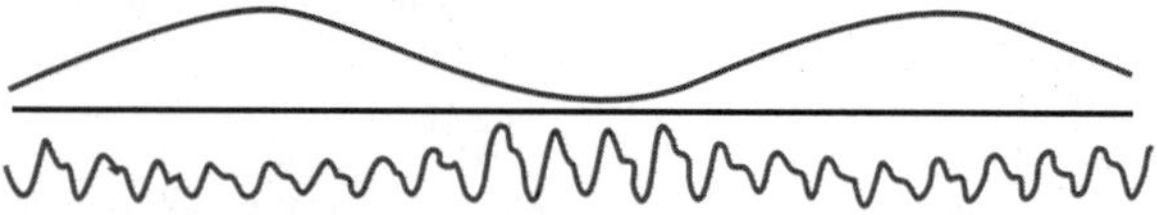

Pulsus Paradoxus
Cardiac tamponade; constrictive pericarditis

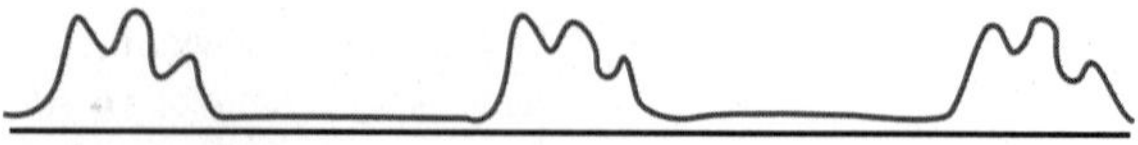

Pulsus Bisferiens
Aortic valve stenosis plus regurgitation

● FIGURE 16-6

Variations in arterial pulses.

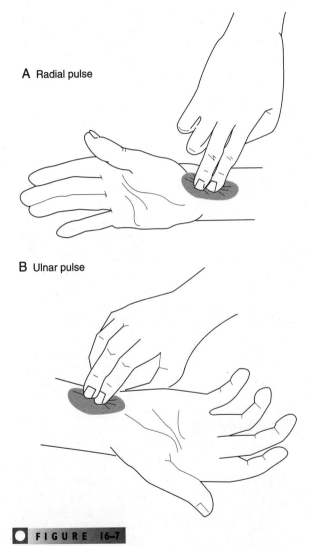

A Radial pulse

B Ulnar pulse

FIGURE 16-7

A, Ulnar pulse. *B*, Radial pulse.

Illustration continued on following page

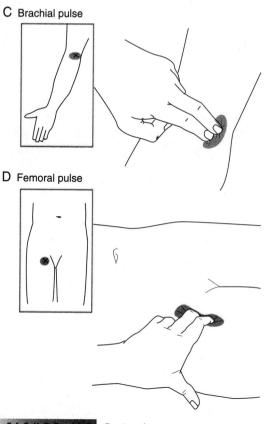

C Brachial pulse

D Femoral pulse

FIGURE 16-7 *Continued*

C, Brachial pulse. *D,* Femoral pulse.

Illustration continued on following page

Popliteal pulse

Palpate the popliteal pulse located behind the knee with the patient supine or prone. Ask the patient to relax the leg muscles and slightly flex the knee (Fig. 16–7*E*).

E Popliteal pulse

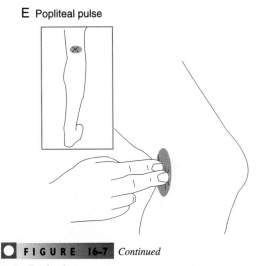

FIGURE 16-7 *Continued*

E, Popliteal pulse.

Illustration continued on following page

Dorsalis pedis pulse	Palpate the dorsalis pedis pulse with the patient supine. It can be found on the anterior or upper aspect of the foot, halfway between the base of the ankle and the second metatarsophalangeal joint (Fig. 16–7*F*).
Posterior tibial pulse	Palpate the posterior tibial pulse just below and behind the medial malleolus with the foot relaxed and slightly extended (Fig. 16–7*G*).

F Dorsalis pulse

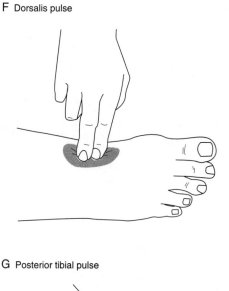

G Posterior tibial pulse

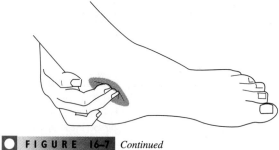

⬤ **F I G U R E   16-7** *Continued*

F, Dorsalis pulse. *G,* Posterior tibial pulse.

Special maneuvers   Allen test: If there are
                         decreased radial or ulnar
                         pulses in the patient's wrist
                         perform the Allen test. Ask the

patient to make a fist and simultaneously obliterate both the ulnar and radial pulses by exerting pressure with your finger tips. Ask the patient to open the fist and release the radial artery. Normally the full palm will become pink. If only half of the palm becomes pink, it is a sign of radial arterial insufficiency. Repeat the test, and this time release only the ulnar artery. Again assess whether there is full or half flushing of the palm. Flushing of half of the palm suggests ulnar arterial insufficiency.

Lower extremities: If there are diminished pulses in the lower extremities perform two special maneuvers. First, with the patient supine, elevate the legs 12 inches off the examining table, and ask the patient to move the feet up and down at the ankles for approximately 1 minute. Note whether extensive pallor occurs. Next, ask the patient to sit up and dangle the legs and feet over the edge of the examining table. Note the whether the pink color returns to the feet, or whether they become dusky red (rubor). Note whether there is a delay in venous return (filling of the veins on top of the feet).

	Normal Findings	Abnormal Findings
Blood pressure	Will vary normally among individuals; in general, systolic pressure 95 to 140 mmHg, diastolic pressure 60 to 90 mmHg (refer to Table Range of Normal Blood Pressure with Respect to Age)	Systolic pressure >140 mmHg or <95 mmHg; diastolic pressure >90 mmHg or <60 mmHg
Sitting	A difference of 5 to 10 mmHg between both arms while sitting	A difference of >10 mmHg in both arms while sitting
Standing	A systolic difference of ≤15 mmHg between both arms; a diastolic difference of ≤5 mmHg between both arms	A systolic difference of >15 mmHg between both arms while standing; a diastolic difference of >5 mmHg between both arms while standing
Orthostatic changes	A difference of <10 mmHg between sitting and standing diastolic BPs taken from the same arm	A difference of >10 mmHg between sitting and standing diastolic pressure taken from the same arm; may indicate orthostatic changes due to blood volume depletion (e.g., GI bleed)
Carotid arteries	A normal rate of 60 to 90 beats/minute	A rate of >60 or >90 beats/minute,

		palpable bilaterally; strong, elastic, and regular; no bruits	an irregular pulse, firm, inelastic, bounding pulse, or a pulse that alternates in strength; change in the rate of the carotid pulse during inspiration (may indicate a sinus dysrhythmia); bruits, a palpable knot, or pulsating mass (requires aggressive work up to rule out thrombosis or aneurysm)
Jugular veins		Jugular venous pressure <1 inch or 2.5 cm	Jugular venous pressure <1 inch or 2.5 cm (sign of heart disease)
Peripheral venous circulation			
Skin			Cyanosis, pallor, rubor or brownish discoloration of the lower extremities (indicates poor circulation or chronic hypoxia); slow healing lesions, ulcers, or necrotic tissue
Temperature		Skin should be warm to touch	The temperature of the extremities is usually normal even with marked venous insufficiency

Pain	No calf tenderness or pain	Tenderness along vein or in calf muscles; aggravated by long periods of standing, sitting, or crossing legs relieved by elevation of the legs, lying down, walking, or use of support hose
Sensation	The patient should be able to perceive soft, sharp, and vibratory sensations	In chronic venous insufficiency, the patient may experience sensory deficits in the extremities
Vessels	Veins appear bluish, feel elastic, and are nontender	Visible areas of reddening or tracking along the course of a vein; palpable tenderness, firm knots, or cords; thick, tortuous vessels; absence of sensation in an area or extremity
Edema	No edema	Edema, usually ascending (beginning in the foot or ankle and progressing to the calf, knee, thigh), is a sign of venous insufficiency
Peripheral arterial circulation		
Skin	Normal skin (refer to Chapter 5, As	Presence of thin, shiny or scaly skin

	(sessment of the Skin, Hair, and Nails)	with decreased hair growth; thickened nails; ulcers on feet or toes that are slow to heal or progress to gangrene and necrosis
Temperature	Extremities are warm to touch; temperature equal in paired extremities	Extremities are cool to touch
Pain	No pain	Tenderness or pain in the extremities, buttocks, calves, or cramps during walking; pain in legs and lower extremities aggravated by exercise and relieved with rest
Sensation	Normal sensation; able to perceive and distinguish light, dull, sharp, and vibratory sensation with eyes closed	Unable to perceive and distinguish light, dull, sharp, and vibratory sensations with eyes closed
Vessels	No bruits	Bruits while auscultating over the aorta, renal, iliac, or femoral arteries (refer to Fig. "Auscultation Landmarks for Detecting Arterial Bruits")
Edema	No edema	Little or no edema

Pulse	All pulses present, strong, elastic, and regular with rating of 1+, 2+, 3+, 4+, etc.	Decreased or absent peripheral pulses
		Bounding pulse: with increased pulse pressure, readily palpable, and not easily obliterated, may be secondary to exercise, anxiety, fever, atherosclerosis, hyperthyroidism
		Pulsus alternans: a pulse that alternates in strength
		Pulsus deferens: the pulses between the left and right extremities are different because of local circulation impairment

Clinical Notes

Be certain to palpate one carotid artery at a time. Use light palpation because increased carotid pressure may stimulate a carotid sinus reflex and lower the heart rate and BP.

Do not overpalpate or massage suspected DVT, as this may inadvertently dislodge the thrombus and cause further harm. A duplex doppler of the lower extremities may be needed to rule out DVT, and if one is present the patient may need anticoagulant therapy.

If the patient has marked edema of the lower extremities, be certain to assess the patient's respiratory status and rule out congestive heart failure.

Geriatric Considerations

	Normal Findings
Veins	Enlargement, especially in calf veins
Pulses	Palpation of dorsalis pedis and posterior tibial pulses may be more difficult; radial artery may feel stiff, rigid, and tortuous
Orthostatic BP	Common in advanced age as a result of a decline in barore-ceptor sensitivity

Clinical Notes

Falls can result from orthostatic BP changes. Carefully assess and communicate these changes to other health care professionals.

Pediatric Considerations

Normal Findings	*Common Variations*	*Abnormal Findings*
Newborn		
Deep red, ruddy coloring	Acrocyanosis	
	Hands and feet cool to touch	
Infant	Generalized mottling	

17

Assessment
of the
Abdomen

HISTORY AND CURRENT
STATUS QUESTIONS

Personal history

Past history of liver, gallbladder, kidney, or gastrointestinal (GI) diseases such as cirrhosis, hepatitis, gallstones, renal stones, pyelonephritis, frequent urinary tract infections (UTIs), peptic ulcer disease, hiatal hernia (HH), diverticulosis, colitis, Crohn's disease, irritable bowel syndrome, or cancer (CA); history of GI bleeding (source, transfusions, surgery); alcohol consumption (amount per day)

Family history

Family members with any of the problems listed above; alcohol consumption by family members

Pain?

Evaluate all complaints of pain for provocative/palliative fac-

QUADRANT METHOD

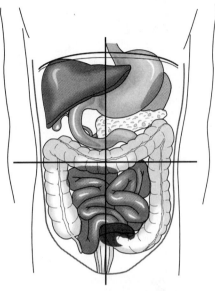

RIGHT UPPER QUADRANT (RUQ)	LEFT UPPER QUADRANT (LUQ)
Liver and gallbladder	Left liver lobe
Pylorus	Stomach
Duodenum	
Head of pancreas	Body of pancreas
Hepatic flexure of colon	Splenic flexure of colon
Portions of ascending and transverse colon	Portions of ascending and transverse colon

RIGHT LOWER QUADRANT (RLQ)	LEFT LOWER QUADRANT (LLQ)
Cecum and appendix	Sigmoid colon
Portion of ascending colon	Portion of descending colon

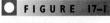

FIGURE 17-1

Abdominal quadrants.

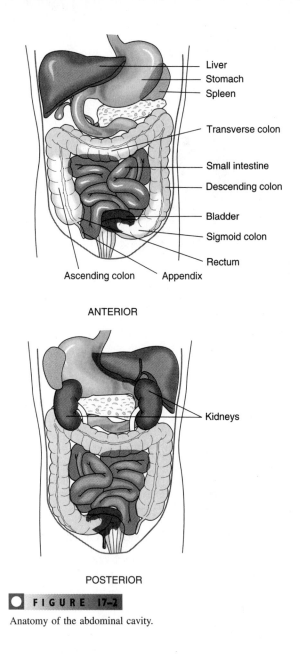

Liver
Stomach
Spleen

Transverse colon

Small intestine
Descending colon

Bladder

Sigmoid colon

Rectum

Ascending colon   Appendix

ANTERIOR

Kidneys

POSTERIOR

FIGURE 17-2

Anatomy of the abdominal cavity.

tors, quality, region, severity, and timing (PQRST Chapter 15, Fig. 15–2); location of the pain (referring to the four quadrants of the abdomen formed by two imaginary perpendicular lines running through the umbilicus) (see Fig. 17–1)

Change in bowel habits?

Last bowel movement; change in frequency of bowel movements; constipation, straining, and difficulty moving bowels; diarrhea or urgency on moving bowels; change in the color (yellow, gray, black, blood streaked), consistency (hard, loose, watery, greasy), or shape (pencil thin or pipe stemmed) of the stool

Flatulence?

Increased belching or flatulence; diet high in gas-producing foods (onions, cabbage, carbonated beverages)

Nausea or vomiting?

Frequency, time of day, associated with eating; any food kept down without vomiting; bile, coffee grounds appearance, or hematemesis

Genitourinary symptoms?

Difficulty initiating a stream of urine, change in frequency of urination, urgency, dysuria, hematuria, pyuria, polyuria, oliguria, nocturia, leaking urine, incontinence, or stress incontinence, passage of a ureteral stone, penile or vaginal discharge?

Dysphagia?	Inability to swallow solids, liquids; frequent regurgitation after eating; bolus sensation in the throat after eating
Change in appetite?	Excessive hunger or lack of appetite (over what period of time), associated weight change
Change in weight?	Significant change in weight (how much, over what period of time)
Increasing abdominal girth?	Marked change in body habitus (increasing abdominal girth, pregnancy, ascites, tumor, impaction)
Decreased activity?	Hospitalized, wheelchair bound, depressed
Medications?	Aspirin or nonsteroidal anti-inflammatories; overuse of laxatives; narcotics, phenothiazines, iron, or any medications that may have increasing or decreasing bowel motility as a side effect

PHYSICAL EXAMINATION

Equipment

Stethoscope
Tape measure

Procedures, Techniques, and Findings

Procedure

Technique

1. Prepare the patient for the exam.

Ask the patient to undress to the waist and lie supine with knees slightly flexed and arms at the side or folded across the chest (you may need to provide pillows for the head and knees to make the patient more comfortable). Drape the upper chest to the xiphoid process and the legs and genitalia up to the symphysis pubis. Ask the patient to locate any tender areas before proceeding and examine these areas last. Examine the patient with warm hands and a warm stethoscope, distracting the patient with conversation while watching his facial expressions for confirmation of pain.

2. Observe the patient's posture.

Note whether the patient is guarding or splinting the abdomen, lying perfectly still, constantly changing position, or favoring one side or position.

3. Inspect the skin.

Note the color of the skin, turgor, and presence of erythema, ecchymosis, lesions, masses, striae, old scars, or venous abnormalities (refer to Chapter 6, Assessment of the Skin, Hair, and Nails).

4. Inspect the abdomen.

Inspect the abdomen from all angles while the patient is lying supine and again while the patient holds a deep breath. Note the symmetry, the contour (flat, convex, or concave), the presence of surface movements (breathing, peristalsis, aortic pulsations), bulging or masses (hernias, cysts, tumors), obesity, and distension (obstruction, ascites) (see Fig. 17–11).

5. Auscultate for bowel sounds.

Using the diaphragm of the stethoscope, auscultate the abdomen in all four quadrants formed by two imaginary lines running perpendicularly through the umbilicus (see Fig. 17–1). Begin in the left lower quadrant (LLQ) and listen for a full 5 minutes. If bowel sounds are present note their character and frequency and whether they are normal, hyperactive, or hypoactive. If they are absent, make note of this, and proceed to the other three quadrants, again auscultating in each for a full 5 minutes.

6. Auscultate for abdominal bruits.

Using the bell of the stethoscope, auscultate for abdominal bruits in the target areas diagrammed (Fig. 17–3). Listen carefully for bruits, venous hums, and friction rubs in the epigastric area and all four quadrants over the aortic, renal, iliac, and femoral arteries and the thoracic aorta. If bruits are present, notify the physician of record and do not palpate the abdomen, as this may damage an existing aneurysm.

7. Percuss the abdomen.

Using the percussion technique (see Chapter 2, Fig. 2–3), percuss all four quadrants of the abdomen to determine the na-

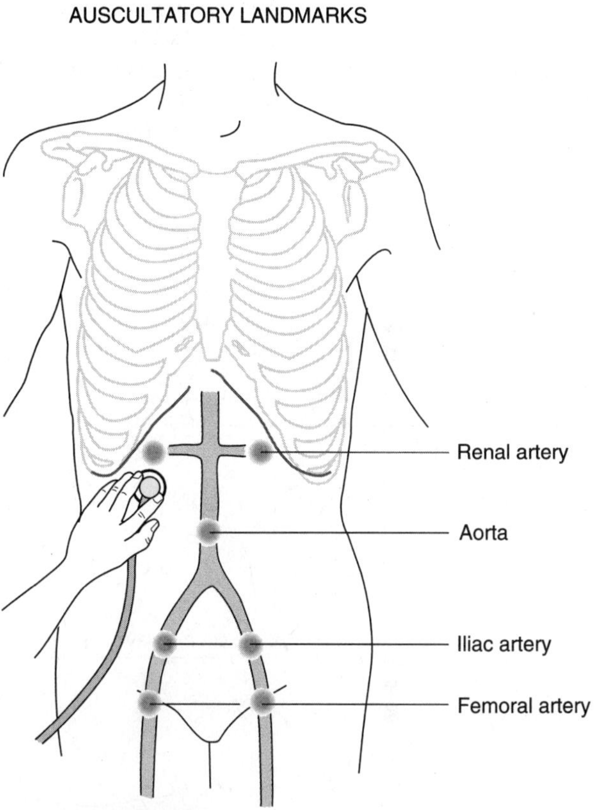

AUSCULTATORY LANDMARKS

Renal artery

Aorta

Iliac artery

Femoral artery

FIGURE 17–3

Auscultation for abdominal bruits.

ture of underlying tissue. Hollow organs (such as the gastric air bubble in the left upper quadrant, LUQ) will produce tympanic sounds, and solid or fluid-filled tissue (such as the liver, kidneys, spleen, pancreas, and distended bladder) will produce a dull sound.

8. Percuss the size and span of the liver.

Percuss upward to the lower liver edge from a point just below the umbilicus on the right midclavicular line. Mark the area where the dullness of the lower liver edge begins. Per-

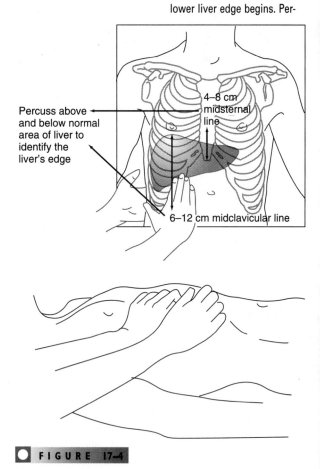

Percuss above and below normal area of liver to identify the liver's edge

4–8 cm midsternal line

6–12 cm midclavicular line

FIGURE 17-4

Measurement of the liver span.

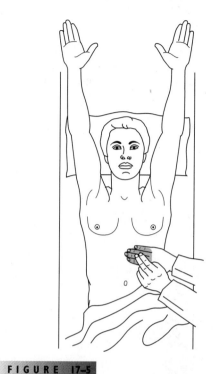

FIGURE 17-5

Percussion of the gastric air bubble.

cuss downward to the upper liver edge from an area of resonant lung. Mark the area where the dullness of the upper liver edge begins. Measure between the two marks with a ruler or tape measure. This measure is the liver span (Fig. 17–4).

9. Percuss the gastric air bubble.

Percuss over the LUQ, the left anterior rib cage, and left epigastric area for the gastric air bubble. It will produce tympany in a small area of the LUQ (Fig. 17–5).

10. Percuss the kidneys.

Ask the patient to sit or stand and percuss the posterior costovertebral angle (CVA) at the scapular line. Painless dullness should be produced over both kidneys (Fig. 17–6).

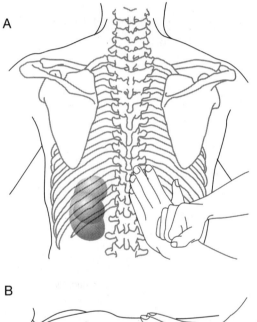

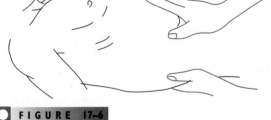

FIGURE 17–6

A, Percussion of kidneys. *B,* Palpalion of kidneys.

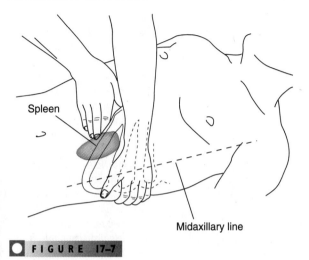

Spleen

Midaxillary line

FIGURE 17-7

Percussion of the spleen.

11. Percuss the spleen.	Percuss in the area of the left 10th rib just posterior to the midaxillary line. Identify the small oval area of splenic dullness. You may also percuss the normally tympanic area in lowest left interspace on the anterior axillary line. If this tympanic area grows dull when the patient takes a deep breath, the spleen may be enlarged (Fig. 17-7).
12. Palpate the abdomen in all four quadrants using the technique of light palpation (see Chapter 2, Fig. 2-1).	Lightly palpate the four quadrants of the abdomen to relax the patient and identify underlying organs, superficial lesions, masses, adipose tissue, and areas of increased resistance or tenderness. Pal-

pate the abdomen with the patient supine, and again with the head slightly lifted. Use the fingerpads or palmar surface of three or four fingers held together. Move methodically through each quadrant, depressing the abdomen not more than ½ to 1 inch, while using dipping or circular motions. Note the size, location, and nature of any perceived abnormalities. Further evaluate any areas of increased resistance while deliberately distracting the patient to determine whether the resistance is voluntary or involuntary. Palpate for rigidity of the rectus muscles that persists despite all techniques of relaxation.

13. Palpate the abdomen in all four quadrants using the technique of deep palpation (see Chapter 2, Figs. 2–2*A,B*). (Do not palpate deeply if tenderness was noted on light palpation.)

Using the palmar surface or fingerpads of three or four fingers held together, deeply palpate the abdomen, depressing tissue 1 to 3 inches as you move methodically through each quadrant. Move your fingers back and forth over underlying tissue to delineate organs and detect less obvious masses. Never palpate over areas of tender pulsating masses, or surgical incisions. If tenderness is elicited, assess for the presence of rebound tenderness, which occurs after the sudden release of deep pressure on the abdomen (Fig. 17–8).

14. Palpate the umbilicus.

Palpate the umbilicus for tenderness, masses, bulges, hernias, lesions, and discharge.

15. Palpate the liver.

Place your left hand under the patient's right posterior thorax parallel to and at the level of the 11th and 12th rib. Place your right hand on the patient's right upper quadrant (RUQ) over the midclavicular line with fingers pointing toward the head and positioned below the lower edge of liver dullness. Ask the patient to take a deep breath while pressing inward and upward with the fingers of

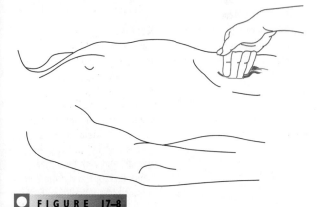

● **FIGURE 17–8**

Deep pressure on the abdomen.

your right hand. Attempt to feel
the liver edge as it descends
(see Fig. 17–4).

16. Palpate the gallbladder.

Ask the patient to take a deep
breath and palpate deep below
the liver margin for enlargement of the gallbladder (see
Fig. 17–4) (which is normally
not palpable).

17. Palpate the spleen.

Place your left hand under the
patient's left CVA and your
right hand on the abdomen below the left costal margin. Ask
the patient to take a deep
breath while you press the fingertips of your right hand inward. Palpate the edge of the
spleen as it descends with
inspiration (see Fig. 17–7).

18. Palpate the aorta.

Use your thumb and forefinger
to palpate the aorta by pressing deeply just to the left of
the verticle midline of the
abdomen.

19. Palpate for ascites
if the abdomen
appears distended.

Ask the patient to lie supine.
Have a colleague assist you by
pressing his hand and forearm firmly along the vertical
midline of the abdomen. Place
your hands on either side of
the patient's abdomen. Strike
one side of the patient's abdomen forcefully with your fingertips, and with the other
hand, feel for the rebounding
impulse of a fluid wave (Fig.
17–9A). Another technique for
determining the presence of

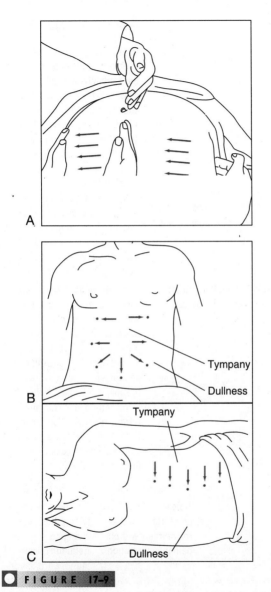

FIGURE 17–9

A, Test for fluid wave. *B,* Test for shifting dullness (supine). *C,* Test for shifting dullness (lying on side).

ascites is to percuss "shifting dullness" in the abdomen. With the patient lying supine, percuss from the midline of the abdomen to the flank (Fig. 17–9*B*). Mark the level of dullness. Ask the patient to lie on his side and percuss again over the same area, this time from the flank to the vertical midline of the abdomen. Note any change in the level of dullness. If ascites is present, the level of dullness will be slightly higher with the patient lying on his side (Fig. 17–9*C*).

20. Perform ballottement for any suspected masses.

It may be difficult to palpate a suspected mass in a patient who has significant ascites. In this situation, ballottement may prove helpful. Thrust the fingers of the right hand suddenly and forcefully into the area of the suspected mass. If the mass is freely mobile, it will initially retreat into the abdomen and immediately rebound back upward against the examiner's fingers (Fig. 17–10).

	Normal Findings	*Abnormal Findings*
Posture	Able to sit or lie comfortably and to move freely without pain in any position	Guarding, splinting, lying perfectly still, changing position frequently, leaning forward, favoring side or position
Skin	Color consistent with the rest of the	Presence of erythema, ecchy-

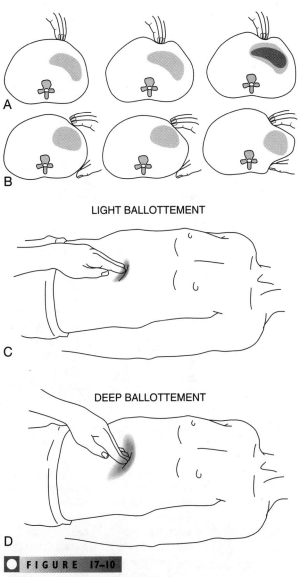

LIGHT BALLOTTEMENT

DEEP BALLOTTEMENT

FIGURE 17–10

A, Single-handed ballottement. *B,* Bimanual ballottement. *C,* Light ballottement. *D,* Deep ballottement.

body; skin smooth, supple, without lesions, masses, or venous abnormalities (see Chapter 6, Assessment of the Skin, Hair, and Nails)

mosis, lesions, masses, edema, old surgical scars, venous abnormalities, or markedly diminished or excessive adipose tissue; jaundice, or a yellow hue to the skin and sclera, may indicate underlying liver or gallbladder disease; a glistening taut abdomen may indicate the presence of ascites; a bluish tinge to the abdomen (Cullen's sign) may indicate internal bleeding; bruising of the flank, or Grey Turner's sign, may indicate pancreatitis or internal bleeding

Abdomen

Soft, smooth, consistent, symmetrical, and nontender; flat, convex, or (in thin people) concave; mild distension normally below the umbilicus secondary to a full bladder or stool in the colon; tympany should be

Involuntary guarding, a tender, rigid, or boardlike abdomen, or the presence of rebound tenderness usually indicates an acute process (appendicitis, cholecystitis, pancreatitis, diverticulitis, pelvic in-

percussed over the gastric air bubble and gas-filled bowel; dullness should be percussed over all other underlying organs; light palpation should elicit no tenderness, guarding, or masses; deep palpation may elicit tenderness normally over the xiphoid process, cecum, and sigmoid colon; the abdomen may be symmetrically distended after eating a heavy meal, or in obese patients flammatory disease, ruptured cyst, ruptured ectopic pregnancy, or peritoneal injury); asymmetry above the umbilicus may indicate gastric dilatation, pancreatic cyst, or a malignancy; asymmetry below the umbilicus may indicate pregnancy, fibroid uterus, ovarian cancer, bowel or bladder obstruction, hernias, tumors, or cysts; abnormal distension of the abdomen occurs with the accumulation of fluid, feces, gas, or tumor (as with ascites, bowel obstruction, and cancer) (Fig. 17–11)

A

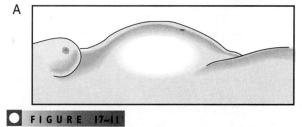

FIGURE 17–11

Abdominal profiles. *A*, Fully rounded or distended, umbilicus inverted.
Illustration continued on following page

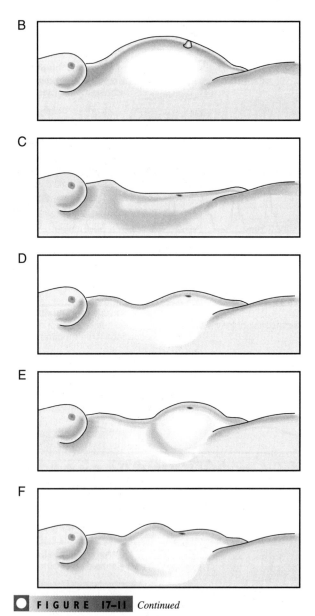

F I G U R E 17–11 *Continued*

B, Distended lower half. *C*, Fully rounded or distended, umbilicus everted. *D*, Distended lower third. *E*, Scaphoid. *F*, Distended upper half.

Bowel sounds	High pitched, irregular gurgling sounds as gas passes through the bowel; singularly or in clusters, last ½ to several seconds, occur at a rate of 1 to 35/minute; normally do not occur in all four quadrants, but should occur in at least one; hyperactive bowel sounds in patients who are hungry or who have just eaten	Hyperactive bowel sounds (borborygmy) in response to inflammation of the bowel, laxative abuse or overuse, and certain spicy foods; Hypoactive bowel sounds or the complete cessation of bowel sounds in response to conditions that decrease the gastric motility such as pancreatitis and paralytic ileus
Bruits	No bruits should be heard	Bruits, venous hums, or friction rubs may indicate an aneurysm, stricture, or thrombosis; *do not palpate the abdomen if bruits are heard,* as this may damage an existing aneurysm
Umbilicus	Free of lesions, masses, hernias, and discharge	An umbilical hernia may cause protrusion or displacement of the umbilicus; tenderness, erythema or discharge may indicate infection or abscess
Stomach	A tympanic area corresponding to	

	the gastric air bubble usually percussed in the left upper quadrant	
Liver	Dull to percussion; span normally 6 to 12 cm (2½ to 5 inches); lower edge often not palpable, however, when palpable, should be smooth, firm, regular, and nontender; liver edge may normally descend up to 1 inch on deep inspiration	Enlarged liver span (>12 cm), irregular contour, or tenderness on deep palpation may indicate cirrhosis, hepatitis, hepatoma, cyst, abscess, or other extrinsic mass or malignancy that impinges on the liver
Gallbladder	Nontender and usually not palpable	Enlarged, palpable, tender gallbladder may indicate cholelithiasis, cholecystitis, malignancy, abscess, or obstruction by an extrinsic mass or malignancy; a positive Murphy's sign, or abrupt cessation of inspiration while deeply palpating the gallbladder, indicative of an acute process
Kidneys	Dull to percussion, not palpable, no CVA tenderness	CVA tenderness may indicate acute pyelonephritis or glomerulonephritis; enlarged, palpable

		kidneys secondary to renal cyst, abscess, or malignancy
Spleen	Dull to percussion, and nontender; not palpable	Change from tympany to dullness while percussing the lowest left interspace as the patient takes a deep breath may indicate an enlarged spleen; enlarged, palpable, or tender spleen
Aorta	Usually palpable (unless the patient is morbidly obese) with strong and regular pulsations	Faint or irregular pulsations may indicate cardiovascular disease; pulsating mass indicates an aneurysm (which should never be further palpated to avoid inflicting damage)

Clinical Notes

Current studies refute past beliefs that analgesics should not be administered to patients with acute abdominal pain prior to physical assessment on the premise that analgesia will mask physical findings. In fact the contrary has been shown to be true, that analgesia has actually helped patients to relax, and has allowed more accurate localization of pain.

Never palpate an abdomen if bruits are present or a pulsating mass has been detected on light palpation. Deep palpation may cause damage to an underlying aneurysm.

Patients presenting with abdominal pain, or alteration in
bowel habits, should be given a digital rectal exam, (refer
to Chapter 20, Assessment of the Anus, Rectum, and
Prostate) and have their stool tested for occult blood.

Special care should be taken when examining pregnant
women to differentiate what may be common symptoms
associated with pregnancy from possible underlying GI
disease.

Some acute conditions of the abdomen (ectopic pregnancy,
ruptured cyst) may produce referred pain to the shoulder.
Patients may present initially with complaints of severe
shoulder pain similar in nature to bursitis.

Geriatric Considerations

	Normal Findings
Abdominal wall	Weakened abdominal muscle tone
	Accumulation of fat in lower abdomen
Bowel sounds	Slowed intestinal motility
Liver	Palpation will be easier

Clinical Notes

Changes attributable to aging often enhance palpation of
abdominal organs. A mass of stool in the descending or
sigmoid colon can be mistaken for malignancy. Treatment
of constipation and reexamination are indicated.

The supine position may be uncomfortable for the older
patient. Place a pillow under the head and knees to
promote comfort.

Pediatric Considerations

Physical Examination

PROCEDURE.

May place child's hand beneath examiner's to reduce tick-
lishness.

Normal Findings	Common Variations	Abnormal Findings
Newborn		
Umbilical cord may fall off in 1 to 2 weeks	Umbilical granuloma	Hard stools
	Umbilical hernia	
	Diastasis recti	
Infant		
Protuberant abdomen		Concave abdomen
Liver edge smooth and palpable 1 to 3 cm below RUQ	Epigastric pulsations	Pyloric stenosis: projectile vomiting, olive-sized mass in RUQ
Spleen tip palpable		
Bladder palpable above symphysis pubis		Intussusception: intermittent pain with current jelly stool
Abdominal breathing pattern		
Child		Hirschprung's disease: megacolon, pencil-thin stools
Protuberant abdomen when erect, flat when supine	Superficial venous pattern	Dilated veins

Clinical Notes

Flexing hips and knees relaxes the abdomen.

Abdominal pain is usually diffuse and general in children, making it difficult to localize inflammation.

Ask child to lift chair in which examiner sits to visualize a hernia.

18

Assessment of the Female Genitalia

HISTORY AND CURRENT STATUS QUESTIONS

Personal sexual history

Sexual orientation (heterosexual, homosexual, bisexual); type of sexual activity engaged in (vaginal, oral, or anal intercourse); frequency of sexual activity; number of partners; "safer sex" practices and condom use; risky practices; previous sexually transmitted diseases (STDs) (when, how treated, tested for cure); recent exposure to a partner with an STD, hepatitis B, or human immunodeficiencey virus (HIV); other risk factors for hepatitis B or HIV; partner tested or treated for either of these

Obstetric history

Note the patient's obstetric history (written G—P_ _ _ _); list in order total number of pregnancies (G), and total number of births, (P) number of premature births, number of abortions (spontaneous and elective combined), and number of living children

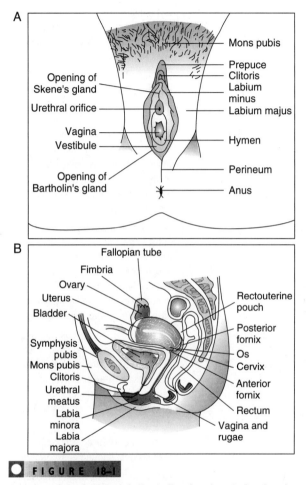

FIGURE 18–1

Anatomy of the female genitalia. *A*, Exterior view. *B*, Interior view.

Menstrual history

Record the patient's menstrual "triad": age of onset of menses, usual number of days duration, and usual length of the menstrual cycle in days; note the LMP, or date of the last menstrual period; note whether the patient reports any premenstrual symptoms of headache, dizziness, cramping, fatigue, anxiety

Menstrual irregularity?

LMP (regular, on time) prior periods regular; missed period (amenorrhea); painful periods (dysmenorrhea), unusually heavy bleeding (menorrhagia), or intermenstrual bleeding or spotting (metrorrhagia); other symptoms associated with menses (headache, fatigue, dizziness, nausea, vomiting, anxiety, premenstrual syndrome)

Pregnancy?

Pain, spotting, discharge, cessation of fetal movement, breast tenderness, nausea, light-headedness, weight change; recent pregnancy test and type (urine or blood, positive or negative); last vaginal intercourse; birth control method used

Birth control?

Method (be as specific as possible, including brand names); past failure problems associated with the use of current or previous methods; recent change of method; known contraindications to any particular method

Pruritis?

Localized or diffuse, location; associated lesions, erythema, excoriations

Infestations?

Lice, scabies, fleas; recent exposure; parasites or nits seen

Lesions?

Type (macule, papule, ulcer, vesicle, rash, laceration, excoriation), number (single or in clusters), location (vulva, labia, vaginal wall, cervix, anus), distribution (symmetrical or

	asymmetrical), pain, pruritis, suppuration
Discharge?	Characteristics (scant, profuse, thick, thin, frothy, malodorous, clear, white, gray, yellow, green); constant or intermittent; relation to the menstrual cycle (during ovulation; prior to, during, or after menses)
Pain?	Type (low abdominal or back pain, diffuse or localized); provocative/palliative factors, quality, region, severity, timing (PQRST) (see Fig. 15–2)
Genitourinary symptoms?	Increased urinary frequency, urgency, dysuria, hematuria, pyuria, polyuria, oliguria, nocturia, incontinence, or stress incontinence; duration of symptoms; associated symptoms (fever, flank pain, abdominal pain, nausea, or vomiting)
Masses or swelling?	Labial edema, Bartholin's cyst or abscess, cystocele, rectocele, uterine prolapse; vulvar, vaginal, cervical cancer; painful or nontender; purulent or draining
Infertility?	Previous pregnancy; time spent "trying" to get pregnant without success; fertility workup (patient and partner), results
Sexual dysfunction?	Loss of libido, loss of orgasm, vaginal atrophy, loss of lubrication, vaginismus, or painful coitus; feelings of ambivalence, insecurity, anxiety, or depression with regard to current relationships
Sexual assault?	Evaluation and counselling by an experienced crisis team

PHYSICAL EXAMINATION

Equipment

Gyn examining table
Gooseneck lamp
Gown
Drape
Gloves
Speculum
Culturettes (both viral and bacterial)
Microscope slides
Normal saline
Potassium hydroxide (KOH)
Papanicoulou (PAP) test scrapers

Procedures, Techniques, and Findings

Procedure	*Technique*
1. Prepare patient and materials for examination.	Ask the patient to urinate and empty her bladder. Have her undress from the waist down and assume a semirecumbent position on the examining table with her knees and thighs draped and her feet in the stirrups. Ask the patient to rest her hands on her waist, relax her knees, and let them fall to the side as far as possible.
2. Inspect and palpate the vulva for lesions, masses, and abnormalities.	Touch the patient's thigh initially to avoid startling her, then proceed with the exam, parting the pubic hair as necessary to facilitate thorough examination. Palpate any noticeable masses, lesions, swelling or abnormalities.

3. Inspect the pubic hair for infestations, density of growth, and sexual maturity.

Part the pubic hair to look for infestations of pubic lice often found at the base of the pubic hair. Search also for nits adhered to the hair stalks. Assess the sexual maturity of the patient (Fig. 18–2).

4. Inspect and palpate the labia majora for lesions, masses, inflammation, swelling, and abnormalities.

Inspect and palpate with one or two fingers any lesions, masses, or abnormalities. You may need to grasp the labia between two fingers to accomplish a thorough examination.

Stage 1
sexual maturity
(preadolescence)

No pubic hair, except for fine body hair

Stage 2
sexual maturity

Sparse growth of long, slightly pigmented, fine pubic hair, which is slightly curly and located along the labia (usually seen at ages 11 to 12)

Stage 3
sexual maturity

Pubic hair becomes darker, curlier, and spreads over the symphysis (usually seen at ages 12 to 13)

Stage 4
sexual maturity

Texture and curl of pubic hair as in adult but not as thick and not spread over the thighs (usually seen between ages 13 & 14)

Stage 5
sexual maturity

Adult appearance in quality of pubic hair; growth is spread onto the inner aspects of the upper thighs

Elderly

Pubic hair is thin, sparse, brittle and gray

FIGURE 18–2

Stages of female sexual maturity.

5. Inspect the labia minora for position, lesions, masses, or abnormalities.

Separate the labia majora with your gloved fingers, and inspect the labia minora for lesions, masses, inflammation, swelling, and abnormalities. Palpate all noticed lesions thoroughly.

6. Inspect the clitoris for position, size, lesions, masses, and abnormalities.

Locate the clitoris between the anterior junction of the labia majora and the labia minora. Inspect and palpate for lesions, masses, enlargement, and abnormalities.

7. Inspect the urethral meatus and Skene's glands for lesions, masses, inflammation, discharge, or abnormalities.

Separate the labia minora and locate the urethral meatus, a small orifice just below the anterior junction of the labia minora. Inspect for lesions, masses, discharge, and abnormalities (Fig. 18–3A). If there is inflammation or urethritis is suspected, milk the urethra gently by inserting a gloved finger into the vagina and stroking its posterior side in a downward motion toward you. Culture any discharge for bacteria, gonorrhea, and chlamydia.

8. Inspect the hymen and note whether it is intact. Inspect the vaginal introitus or vaginal opening for lesions, masses, inflammation, tears, discharge, and support.

Inspect the hymen and vaginal introitus. The hymen may be intact in children and virgins. Inspect for lesions, masses, inflammation, and tears (Fig. 18–3B). Palpate any abnormalities. With the labia separated by your gloved finger, ask the patient to bear down to allow

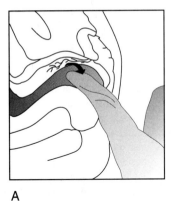

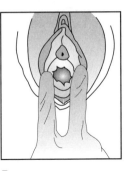

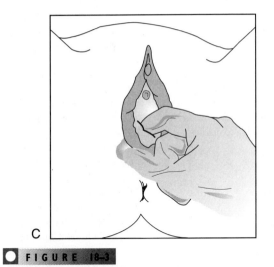

● FIGURE 18-3

Vaginal examination. *A,* Palpation of Skene's glands. *B,* Inspection of hymen and vaginal introitus. *C,* Palpation of Bartholin's glands.

the support of the vaginal outlet to be evaluated. Observe and note any abnormal bulging or swelling.

9. Inspect the Bartholin's glands for pain, swelling, masses, or discharge.

Inspect the Bartholin's glands, located bilaterally at the base of the vaginal opening, for pain, swelling, masses, and discharge (Fig. 18–3C). Palpate the glands between your gloved index finger and your thumb by placing one finger inside the base of the vaginal opening and one on the outside of the labia majora. Gently compress the glands between your two fingers and culture any discharge exuding from the duct openings for bacteria, gonorrhea, and chlamydia.

10. Inspect the cervix and cervical os for position, shape, size, color, inflammation, erythema, lesions, masses, and discharge.

Lubricate your gloved fingers and speculum with water. Insert one or two fingers into the vaginal opening and press downward on the posterior aspect in order to further open the introitus and facilitate the insertion of the speculum. With the speculum closed and held so that the blade width is in a verticle position, insert the speculum. Gently push in a downward sloping fashion, while at the same time rotating the blade so that the width is now in a horizontal position. Follow the vaginal canal to the cervix. Open the speculum and manipulate the cervix into position and secure by clamping (Fig. 18–4). Obtain

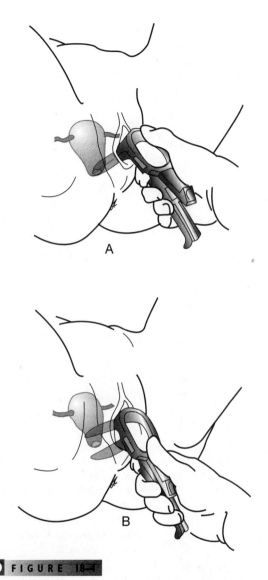

FIGURE 18-4

Vaginal examination. *A,* Insertion of the speculum. *B,* Opening of the speculum blades.

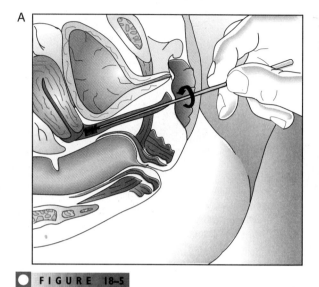

A

FIGURE 18–5

A, Obtaining a cervical smear.

Illustration continued on following page

	specimens for cytology and culture any discharge (Fig. 18–5).
11. Inspect the vaginal outlet for lesions, masses, inflammation, discharge, and abnormalities.	Unclamp the speculum and hold it open as you withdraw it slowly from the vaginal canal. As you withdraw the speculum inspect the walls of the vaginal canal. Use a gooseneck lamp or pen light to better illuminate the canal.
12. Palpate the vaginal wall for masses, lesions, and abnormalities.	Lubricate the index and middle finger of a gloved right hand. Insert the two fingers into the

B

Mycelia and spores
of Candida

Trichomonad

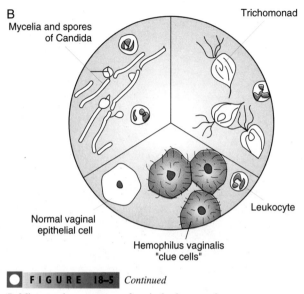

Normal vaginal
epithelial cell

Hemophilus vaginalis
"clue cells"

Leukocyte

○ F I G U R E 18-5 *Continued*

B, Microscopic appearance of vaginal microorganisms.

13. Palpate the cervix for position, shape, size, consistency. Determine whether the cervical os is open or closed.

vagina. Palpate the anterior, posterior, and lateral walls of the vaginal canal.

Palpate the cervix with the tips of your fingers. Note position, shape, consistency, and mobility of the cervix. Gently move the cervix from side to side and test for cervical motion tenderness (Fig. 18–6A). Attempt to admit one fingertip into the cervical os. Usually the os is closed and you will feel tight resistance. If

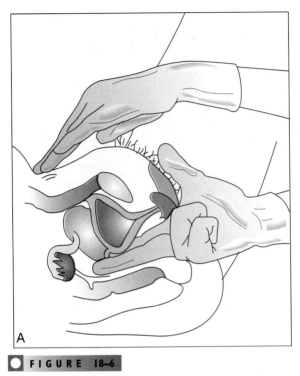

A

FIGURE 18–6

A, Bimanual palpation of the uterus.

Illustration continued on following page

	it admits one fingertip, or offers no resistance, it is considered open.
14. Palpate the ovaries and adnexa.	Place your left hand on the patient's abdomen about halfway between the umbilicus and the symphisis pubis. Push inward and downward toward the symphisis pubis while at the same time pushing upward on the vaginal mucosa lateral

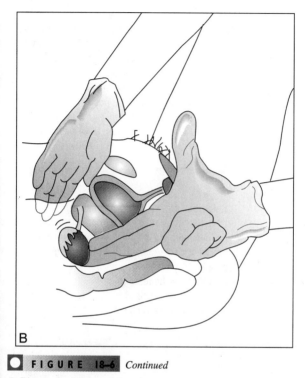

B

● FIGURE 18–6 *Continued*

B, Bimanual palpation of the adnexa.

to the cervix with the fingers of your right hand. Try to palpate the small almond-shaped ovary on either side (Fig. 18–6*B*). Palpate for the adnexa. Normally it will not be palpable unless there is adnexal thickening.

15. Palpate the uterus for position, size, shape, consistency.

With your hands positioned as described above, push downward toward the symphisis pubis with your left hand while pushing upward on the cervix with the fingers of your right hand. Attempt to grasp the uterus between the fingers of your two hands (Fig. 18–6). Note the position, size, shape, consistency, and mobility of the uterus. Note also whether the uterus is tender.

	Normal Findings	*Abnormal Findings*
Vulva		
Skin	Smooth, warm skin; pink in light-skinned people and olive to brown in dark-skinned people, May be lighter in color than the rest of the body because of lack of exposure to sun	Red, hot, erythematous; ecchymosis, hematomas, irregular pigment
Lesions	None	Excoriations, masses, papules, macules, vesicles, ulcers, rash, or wheals
Infestations	None	Lice, scabies, fleas
Pubic hair	Quantity and distribution of pubic hair should be consistent with the sexual maturity expected for the patient's age	Abnormal distribution for age may indicate hormonal imbalances, chronic disease, dermatitis, or response to medication; hair loss may be symmetrical and nonscarring or asymmetrical and scarring

Infestations	None	Lice usually found at the base of the pubic hairs; nits found adhered to the hair stalks
Labia majora	Smooth, moist skin, without lesions, ecchymosis, erythema; usually symmetrical in size and shape; lie together in children and virgins and remain parted open in sexually active women and after childbirth; skin on the inner aspect may be slightly darker	Red, hot, dry, skin; edema, erythema, ecchymosis, tears, lacerations; lesions such as macules, papules, vesicles, ulcers, venereal warts, masses; tenderness
Clitoris	Normally pink without lesions; size does not exceed 2 cm in length by 0.5 cm in width	Bright red color, erythema, ecchymosis, lesions; enlarged clitoris may indicate hormonal or developmental masculinization; may also be excised in some religious and cultural groups
Urethral meatus	Located midline and anterior to the vaginal opening; pink with a slitlike opening; without lesions, discharge, tenderness	Red, erythematous; prolapse, polyps, fistula, lesions, discharge, edema, tenderness
Hymen	May be intact in virgins and restrict the opening of the vagina; in sexually active women only remnants of the hymen remain	If edematous, torn, or absent in small children sexual abuse must be considered

Introitus	Usually open and un-obstructed	Obstructed by a cystocele, a bulging mass descending from the anterior vaginal wall, or by a rectocele, arising from the posterior vaginal floor; usually caused by inadequate support of the vaginal outlet; a large smooth pink protruding tissue mass may actually be a uterine prolapse with the cervix visible in the vaginal canal
Bartholin's glands	Normally nontender, and not palpable	Large nontender unilateral mass may be a Bartholin's cyst; a large, hot, tender, fluctuant mass, either unilateral or bilateral may be a Bartholin's abscess; abcess may be fluctuant, have tracked, or have spontaneously ruptured; Discharge from the site may culture positive for gonorrhea, or chlamydia
Vaginal wall	Ruggated homogenous tissue, with thin clear or cloudy odorless secretions; secretions usually increased	Thick, curdlike, or foul-smelling discharge; lesions, masses, vesicles, papules, warts

in pregnancy; no lesions or masses.

Cervix	Usually pink, smooth, moist, glistening, rounded, firm mass, approximately 1 inch in diameter; may be enlarged, soft, and blue tinged in pregnancy, and pale during menopause; os is usually a central depression with a rounded opening in nulliparous women, and a "fish-mouthed" opening in multiparous women; no discharge, lesions, masses, erythema, or cervical motion tenderness are present	Erythema, lesions, discharge, friable surface, bleeding (between periods), lacerations, polyps, prolapse or enlargement of the cervix are abnormal findings; an open cervical os may indicate threatened abortion or incompetent cervix; lesions may indicate STD (papules, venereal warts; vesicles, herpes simplex II; ulcers, either primary syphilis or chancroid; macules, secondary syphilis)
Uterus	Usually firm, nontender, "6-week"-size mass in the nonpregnant female; contour should be smooth, regular, without palpable nodules or masses	Enlarged, soft, or tender; may indicate pregnancy, fibroids, hydatidiform mole, or mass

Clinical Notes

Male practitioners should always be accompanied by a chaperone throughout the course of the examination. Female practitioners should be accompanied by a chaperone if the patient is emotionally unstable.

A thorough gyn exam should include a Pap smear for cytology, cultures for gonorrhea and chlamydia, and a wet prep and KOH for trichomonas and yeast.

A VDRL should be sent on all patients as part of their annual gyn check, and whenever diagnosing or screening for STDs.

A pregnancy test should be sent on all women of childbearing age who complain of vaginal bleeding, low abdominal pain, discharge, or any abnormality of their menstrual cycle.

Choose an appropriate type and size of speculum for the age of patient being examined. Test the clamping device and thumb screws to be sure they are working properly before inserting the speculum into the patient's vagina.

Geriatric Considerations

Normal Findings

Pubic hair	Thin, sparse, and gray
Uterus	Diminished in size
Ovaries	Diminished in size, often not palpable
Labia	Thin, flattened appearance
Vagina	Shorten and narrow in structure; mucosa dry, thin, and pale.

Clinical Notes

A weakening of the pelvic floor musculature may result in protrusion of the bladder (cystocele) or protrusion of the rectum (rectocele) into the vagina.

Dwindling hormones and age-related changes in the pelvic floor and bladder contribute to urge incontinence in the older female patient. Obtain a clear, complete history of voiding patterns.

Pelvic examination in a postmenopausal sexually inactive woman may need to be modified to a single-digit examination.

Pediatric Considerations

History

Bubble baths?
Cotton or other underwear?
Masturbation behaviors?
Known sexual abuse?
Development of secondary sexual characteristics?
Age of menarche? Regular cycle? Dysmenorrhea?
Sexually active? Known to family or confidential?
Knowledge base re: contraception and STDs?
Conflicts re: sexual identity/orientation?

Physical Examination

PROCEDURE. To examine the external genitalia, gently retract the labia; having a small child cough may expose the vaginal mucosa for better visualization.

Normal Findings	Common Variations	Abnormal Findings
Infant		
Labia minora prominent	Edema, bruising of genitals post delivery	Ambiguous genitalia
	Bloody or serosanguinous vaginal discharge	
Infant and Child		
Labia minora atrophy; almost nonexistent until puberty	Perianal skin tags	Vaginal discharge
	Partially fused labia	Near complete fusion of labia obstructing urinary flow
	Secondary sexual characteristics as early as the 8th year	

Clinical Notes

Refer to Tanner staging (see Chapter 13) to determine degree of sexual maturation.

Menstrual cycle may be irregular for 2 years postmenarche.

Secondary amenorrhea for 6 months or less, in the absence of other signs of disease, is of no serious concern in the adolescent.

19

Assessment of the Male Genitalia

HISTORY AND CURRENT STATUS QUESTIONS

Personal sexual history

Sexual orientation (heterosexual, homosexual, bisexual), type of sexual activity engaged in (vaginal, oral, anal intercourse), frequency of sexual activity, number of partners; practices "safer sex" and use condoms; risky practices; past sexually transmitted diseases (STDs) (when treatment, tested for cure); recent exposure to a partner with an STD, hepatitis B, or HIV; other risk factors for hepatitis B or HIV, tested or treated for either of these

Pruritus?

Type (local or diffuse; groin, penis, scrotum, thighs, anus, buttocks); association with a rash, lesions, erythema; use of over-the-counter medications (what brand, provide relief)

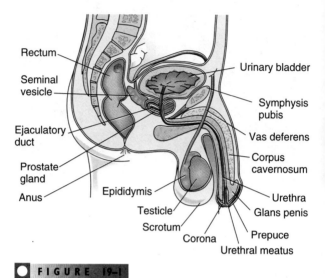

Anatomy of the male genitalia.

Infestations?	Lice, scabies, or fleas; recent exposure; parasites or nits seen; prior treatment; over-treatment (e.g., lindane toxicity from overzealous delousing)
Lesions?	Type (macule, papule, ulcer, vesicle, rash, laceration, excoriation), amount (single or clustered), location (groin, penis, scrotum, thighs, anus), distribution (symmetrical, asymmetrical, along a dermatome, involving more than one dermatome), pain, pruritis, suppuration
Discharge?	Character (scant, profuse; thick, thin; malodorous; clear, white, gray, yellow, green,

	blood tinged; constant or intermittent) association with urination or ejaculation
Pain?	Type (local or diffuse); location (groin, penis, scrotum, thighs, anus); trauma to the groin or genitals, provocative/palliative factors, quality, region, severity, and timing (see Fig. 15–2)
Genitourinary symptoms?	Difficulty initiating stream of urine, change in frequency of urination, urgency, dysuria, hematuria, pyuria, polyuria, oliguria, nocturia, leaking urine, incontinence, or stress incontinence; how long; associated symptoms (fever, malaise, flank pain, abdominal pain, nausea, or vomiting); history of benign prostatic hypertrophy (BPH), prostatitis, renal or urethral calculi
Masses or swelling?	Location (groin, inguinal area, penis, scrotum, thighs, anus); characteristics (tender or nontender; soft or hard; fluctuant or draining) how long has it been there; change in size over time
Infertility?	Past conception; time spent "trying" without success; infertility work-up (patient, partner), results
Sexual dysfunction?	Loss of libido, inability to have an erection, to climax, to ejaculate; premature ejac-

ulation; painful coitus; feelings
of ambivalence, insecurity,
anxiety, or depression with regard to current relationships

Sexual abuse or assault?   recent or remote sexual abuse
or assault; evaluation and
counselling by an experienced
crisis team

PHYSICAL EXAMINATION

Equipment

Gloves
Reflex hammer
Materials for genital cultures

Procedures, Techniques, and Findings

Procedure

Technique

1. Inspect the external genitalia and assess sexual
   maturity.

Note the distribution of pubic
hair (absent in infants and children and thick, extending onto
thighs, in adults). Note the
shape and size of the penis
(usually adult size and shape
after puberty). Note size, color,
and texture of scrotum (darkened and ruggated after puberty). Assess for sexual maturity (Fig. 19–2).

2. Inspect and palpate the skin
   for color, temperature, lesions, masses, excoriations,
   lacerations, abnormalities,
   infestations, or lack of
   hygiene.

Part the pubic hair as necessary to facilitate thorough examination. Gently move and
manipulate the penis and scrotum to allow visualization of
their posterior sides. Palpate
thoroughly and note the type
and location of any noticed lesions (macules, papules, ul-

	Pubic hair	Penis	Testes and scrotum
Stage 1 **Sexual maturity**	None except for fine body hair as on the abdomen	Size proportional to body size as in childhood	Size proportional to body size as in childhood
Stage 2 **Sexual maturity**	Sparse, long, slightly pigmented, thin hair at the base of the penis	Slight enlargement	Enlargement of testes and scrotum; reddened pigmentation; texture more prominent
Stage 3 **Sexual maturity**	Darkens, becomes more coarse and curly; growth extends over symphysis	Elongation	Enlargement continues
Stage 4 **Sexual maturity**	Continues to darken, thicken, and become coarser and more curly; growth extends	Breadth and length increase; glans develops	Enlargement continues; skin pigmentation darkens
Stage 5 **Sexual maturity**	Adult distribution and appearance; growth extends to inner thighs	Adult appearance	Adult appearance
Elderly clients	Hair sparse and gray	Decrease in size	Testes hang low in scrotum; scrotum appears pendulous

⬤ **F I G U R E 19-2**

Stages of sexual maturity.

cers, vesicles, rash, laceration, excoriation, mass).

3. Inspect and palpate the pre-puce or foreskin in uncir-cumcised males.

Note any lesions, swelling, edema, lacerations, erythema, or ecchymosis. Gently retract the foreskin. Inspect the interior. Pay particular atten-tion to the junction between the prepuce and the glans, as this is often the preferred site of STD-related lesions.

4. Inspect and palpate the glans.

Inspect and palpate the full surface of the glans, noting exact location of any lesions, masses, swelling, edema, ab-normalities, erythema, or ec-chymosis. The glans will be moist and pink in uncircum-cised males, and appear more reddish and dry in cir-cumcised males.

5. Inspect the urethral meatus for position, abnormalities, and discharge.

Note the location of the urinary meatus and check for hypospa-dias (abnormal position of the meatus, usually on posterior side). Note location and type of lesions or abnormalities. In-spect for prolapse, fissures, and fistulas. Gently compress the glans between your thumb and finger (or allow patient to do this) to open the meatus slightly (Fig. 19–3B). Inspect the color and discharge. Culture any discharge present for gon-orrhea, chlamydia, and bacte-ria. You may also want to do a potassium hydroxide (KOH) and wet prep to look for yeast and trichomonas at this time. (Note: If the patient complains of discharge and none is seen, you may need to milk the shaft of the penis gently to produce a bead of discharge.)

6. Inspect and palpate the shaft of the penis.

Gently manipulate and lift the penis to allow inspection and palpation of the entire surface area. Note exact location and type of lesions, masses, or abnormalities. Palpate for induration and tenderness along the ventral surface (Fig. 19–3A). In infants and children this may be omitted.

7. Inspect and palpate the scrotum and testes for size, shape, color, temperature, tenderness, lesions, abnormalities.

Gently palpate the testicles by grasping them between your thumb and forefinger (Fig. 19–3C). Palpate the epididymis, spermatic cord, and vas deferens. Note any lesions, masses, tenderness, or enlargement. Illuminate the scrotum and testicle if a mass is suspected or an enlargement is observed. A fluid-filled mass will illuminate well, while a mass filled with blood, pus, or solid tissue will not.

8. Inspect and palpate for hernias.

Ask the patient to stand and bear down as though having a bowel movement. Inspect the inguinal areas and scrotum for any bulging or masses. With one finger, press inward on the loose skin at a low point on the scrotum. Follow the spermatic cord upward by invaginating

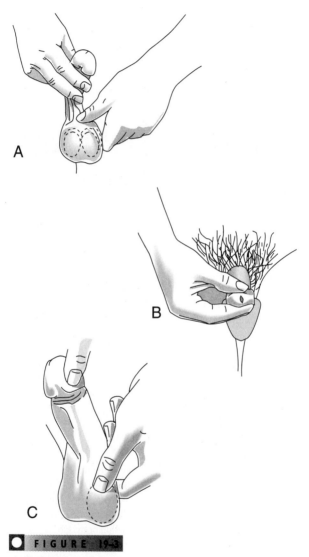

A, Examination of penis and scrotum. *B,* Examination of urethral meatus. *C,* Examination of spermatic cord and testes.

loose scrotal skin until you can palpate the external inguinal ring. If possible, follow the inguinal canal to the internal inguinal ring. Ask the patient to bear down and again feel for any bulging or masses. If a hernia is palpated, apply gentle pressure and note whether it is reducible. (Never force your finger into the inguinal canal. If you meet with resistance, or the patient complains of pain stop the exam.)

9. Palpate the prostate gland.   See Chapter 20, Assessment of the Anus, Rectum, and Prostate.

	Normal Findings	*Abnormal Findings*
Skin	Warm, smooth skin without lesions, ecchymosis, erythema	Hot, red skin indicates cellulitis or inflammation; presence of lesions may indicate dermatitis or venereal disease (macules, secondary syphilis; papules, venereal warts; ulcers, syphilis; vesicles, herpes simplex II; excoriations, lice or scabies; rash, candidiasis)
Pubic hair	Density of growth and distribution should be consistent with that	Abnormal quantity and distribution for age may indicate hormonal im-

	expected for patient's age group	balances, chronic disease, dermatitis or response to medications; hair loss may be symmetrical and nonscarring, or asymmetrical and scarring
Prepuce	Normally without lesions, lacerations, edema; easily retractable; smegma, a whitish pasty exudate, may normally be present	Presence of lesions, lacerations, edema, erythema; inability to retract the prepuce (phimosis) or inability to replace a retracted prepuce (paraphimosis) are abnormal and indicate disease
Glans	Appears pink and moist in uncircumcised males, and may appear dry and reddish in circumcised males; no lesions, masses, erythema, ecchymosis	Presence of any lesions or masses as described above; balanitis, or inflammation of the glans with marked erythema; edema
Urethral meatus	A pink, slitlike opening located in the center of the glans; no lesions, masses, or discharge	Hypospadias, or congenital displacement of the urethral meatus (usually on posterior portion of the glans or shaft); urethral prolapse (a perceivable small rosette of prolapsed

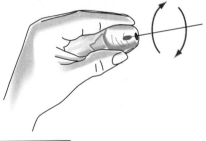

⬤ FIGURE 19–4

Culturing genital discharge in the male.

		membranes protruding from the meatus); discharge (clear, yellow, white, or blood-tinged) may indicate urethritis and must be cultured and treated appropriately (Fig. 19–4)
Shaft	No lesions, erythema, ecchymosis, edema	Presence of any lesions as described above may indicate venereal disease; tenderness or induration along the ventral surface may indicate urethral stricture and periurethral inflammation, or carcinoma
Scrotum and testes	Coarse, loose, ruggated skin of slightly darker pig	Undescended testes; cryptorchidism or poorly de-

ment than the rest of the body; no lesions, erythema, edema, masses, or swelling; sensitive, but not painful, to gentle compression between two fingers; not >1 inch diameter in size; Left testis is normally lower than the right

veloped scrotum on one or both sides; presence of lesions, masses, edema, erythema, ecchymosis

Nontender swelling or mass:

Hydrocele/ spermatocele: fluid-filled cysts of the tunica vaginalis and epididymis that transilluminate

Testicular cancer: a hard, palpable nodule usually on anterior side of the testis

Tender swelling or mass:

Scrotal edema: from chronic exacerbated congestive heart failure, chronic renal failure, or nephrotic syndrome

Epididymitis: acute bacterial infection of epididymis. May be accompanied by urethritis and discharge

		Testicular torsion: occasionally torsion of
Vas deferens and spermatic cord	No masses, thickening, or tenderness	Any swelling, mass, or tenderness
		Varicocele: bead-like nodules or varicosities (bag of worms) palpated usually on the left side
		Thickening of the vas deferens or spermatic cord may occur with chronic infections and tuberculosis
Hernias	None	Direct inguinal hernia: palpated above the inguinal ligament close to the external inguinal ring; it bulges anteriorly, does not travel down the inguinal canal, and may, but rarely does, invade the scrotum
		Indirect inguinal hernia: palpated above the inguinal ligament close to the internal inguinal ring; it travels down the

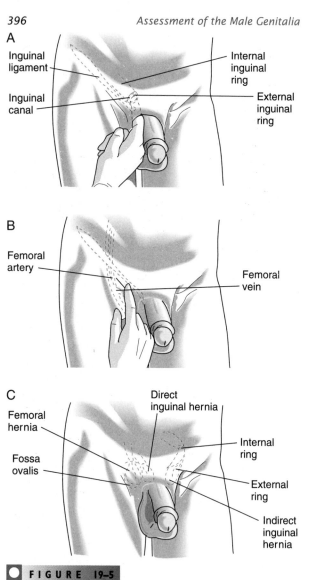

A, Inguinal ligament, Inguinal canal, Internal inguinal ring, External inguinal ring

B, Femoral artery, Femoral vein

C, Direct inguinal hernia, Femoral hernia, Fossa ovalis, Internal ring, External ring, Indirect inguinal hernia

● FIGURE 19–5

A, Palpation for inguinal hernia. *B*, Palpation for femoral hernia. *C*, Comparative locations of direct inguinal, indirect inguinal, and femoral hernias.

inguinal canal and
often invades the
scrotum

Femoral hernia: pal-
pated below the
inguinal ligament
and appears more
lateral than inguinal
hernias; difficult to
distinguish from
enlarged inguinal
lymph nodes

All hernias may be-
come painful if
strangulation oc-
curs, either by tor-
sion of bowel or
compression by
surrounding tissue
(Fig. 19–5).

Clinical Notes

Palpate external genitalia gently so as not to cause the patient undue embarrassment by stimulating an erection.

Never force your finger into the inguinal canal. If you are
met with firm resistance or the patient complains of pain,
stop the examination.

Testicular torsion is a surgical emergency. If suspected, the
patient must receive immediate attention to prevent the
necrosis of a testis.

Patients should be instructed in the techniques of testicular
self-examination.

Geriatric Considerations

Normal Findings:

Pubic hair   Thin, sparse, gray

Testes   Less firm, smaller in size, skin

less taut, resulting in a more
pendulous appearance

Penis   Decrease in size

Clinical Notes

Size changes do not mean a change in libido or function. Most older men remain sexually active.

Pediatric Considerations

History

Masturbatory behaviors?
Known sexual abuse?
Development of secondary sexual characteristics?
Sexually active? Known to family or confidential?
Knowledge base re: contraception and STDs?
Conflicts re: sexual identity/orientation?

Penile epispadias

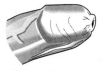

Phimois

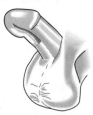

Penile hypospadias

Paraphimosis

● FIGURE 19–6

Abnormalities of male genitalia.

TABLE 19–1
Common Abnormalities of the Male Genitalia

Abnormality	Definition/causation	Basis for diagnosis
Hydrocele	An accumulation of serous fluid between the visceral and parietal layers of the tunica vaginalis	Transilluminates; fingers can get above the mass
Scrotal hernia	A hernia within the scrotum	Bowel sounds auscultated; does not transilluminate; fingers cannot get above the mass
Varicocele	Abnormal dilatation and tortuosity of the veins of the pampiniform plexus; often described as a "bag of worms" in the scrotum	Complaints of a dragging sensation or dull pain in the scrotal area; feels like a soft bag of worms; collapses when the scrotum is elevated and increases when the scrotum is dependent; more commonly appears on the left side; usually appears at puberty

Table continued on following page

TABLE 19–1
Common Abnormalities of the Male Genitalia *Continued*

Abnormality	Definition/causation	Basis for diagnosis
Spermatocele	An epididymal cyst resulting from a partial obstruction of the spermatic tubules	Transilluminates; round mass, feels like a third testis; painless
Tuberculosis	May be a result of benign or malignant neoplasms, syphilis, or tuberculosis	Nodules are not tender; in tuberculosis lesions, vas deferens often feels beaded
Epididymitis	An inflammation of the epididymis, usually resulting from *Escherichia coli*, *Neisseria gonorrhoeae*, or *Mycobacterium tuberculosis* organisms	Spermatic cord often thickened and indurated; pain relieved by elevation

Table continued on following page

T A B L E   19–1
Common Abnormalities of the Male Genitalia *Continued*

Abnormality	Definition/causation	Basis for diagnosis
Torsion of the spermatic cord	Axial rotation or volvulus of the spermatic cord, resulting in infarction of the testicle	Elevated mass; pain not relieved by further elevation; more common in childhood or adolescence; history of extreme pain and tenderness of the testis, followed by hyperemic swelling and hydrocele
Testicular tumor	Multiple causes	Usually not painful; hydroceles may develop as a result of a tumor— if a testis cannot be palpated, fluid need to be aspirated so that the testes can be accurately evaluated

Normal Findings	*Common Variations*	*Abnormal Findings (Fig. 19–6, Table 19–1)*
Newborn and Infant		
Foreskin adheres to glans penis	Edema, bruising of the genitals post-delivery	Hypospadias: meatus located along ventral surface of glans or shaft of penis; foreskin incomplete
Testes in scrotum	Testes in inguinal canal, can be milked down into scrotum	Undescended testicle
	Hydrocele: scrotum transilluminates	
		Hernias: inguinal or scrotal mass

Child

Foreskin retractable

Clinical Notes

Refer to Fig. 19–2 to determine degree of sexual maturation.

20

Assessment of the Anus, Rectum, and Prostate

HISTORY AND CURRENT STATUS QUESTIONS

Pruritus?	Rash; lice, scabies, or pinworms
Lesions?	Type (macules, papules, ulcers, vesicles, excoriations, lacerations), location, length of time present, tender or nontender, exudate, obstruction of the anus, interference with normal defecation and hygiene
Abdominal distension or mass?	Internal or external hemorrhoids, prolapsed rectum, rectal mass or cancer, perianal abcess, palpable or enlarged inguinal nodes, distension of the abdomen or palpable abdominal masses (evidence of obstruction or urinary retention)
Flatulence?	Diet high in gas-producing

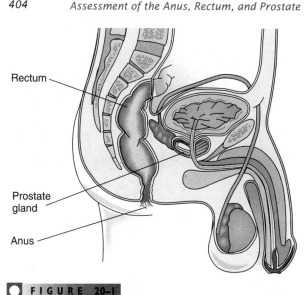

FIGURE 20–1

Anal canal, rectum, and prostate.

	foods (onions, cabbage, carbonated drinks)
Diet?	Diet high in fat or low in fiber
Bowel habits?	Diarrhea, constipation, urgency, frequency, nocturnal defecation, incontinence of stool, blood or mucus in the stool; characteristics of stool brown, yellow, gray, black; watery, loose, formed, greasy, hard; pencil, ribbon, or pipe-stemmed stool
Genitourinary symptoms?	Difficulty initiating a stream of urine, change in frequency of urination, urgency, dysuria, hematuria, pyuria, polyuria, oli-

guria, nocturia, leaking urine, stress incontinence, or incontinence; duration of symptoms; associated symptoms (fever, malaise, flank pain, abdominal pain, nausea, or vomiting); history of benign prostatic hypertrophy (BPH), prostatitis, renal or ureteral calculi

Pain?

Palliative/provocative factors, quality, region, severity, timing (PQRST), type (low back, low abdominal, rectal, anal) association with defecation (concomitant, increase) (see Fig. 15–2)

PHYSICAL EXAMINATION

Equipment

Gloves
Hemoccult card test solution

Procedures, Techniques, and Findings

Procedure	*Technique*
1. Inspect and palpate perianal tissue and perineum.	If the rectal exam is to be performed at the end of a gyn exam, the patient may remain in the semirecumbent or lithotomy position; otherwise, position the patient (male or female) on the side in the Sims position with knees slightly flexed. Gently retract the buttocks with your gloved hands, and inspect the anal and perianal tissue. Note color, texture, lesions, masses, pro-

	lapse, hemmorrhoids, skin breakdown, etc.
2. Inspect for the appearance of protrusions or masses with straining.	Ask the patient to bear down as though attempting a bowel movement. Inspect for protrusions or masses, including prolapse, polyps, and hemmorrhoids.
3. Perform a digital exam to palpate the anus, rectum, and prostate.	Press gently against the anal sphincter with the gloved and lubricated index fingerpad. Ask patient to bear down and gently press fingertip into the opening of the anus (Fig. 20–2A).
4. Assess the tone and musculature of the anal sphincter.	Palpate the entire surface of the anal sphincter. Ask the patient to tighten the buttocks around your finger to allow assessment of tone and strength of the sphincter.
5. Palpate the muscular anal ring and rectum.	Palpate the entire surface of the muscular anal ring by turning the finger in a circular motion around its own axis. Then move further inward to the rectum and repeat. Note any palpable lesions, masses, lacerations or abnormalities (Fig. 20–2B).
6. Palpate for high masses.	With finger as far into the rectum as possible, ask the patient to bear down and palpate for any descending masses.
7. Palpate prostate in men.	Turn your finger to palpate the anterior rectal wall. Gently palpate the prostate. Try to identify the two lateral lobes and the median sulcus. Note

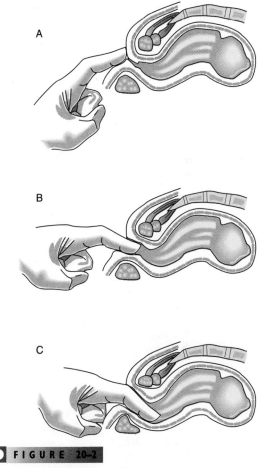

● FIGURE 20-2

Assessment of the rectum and prostate. *A*, Entering the anal opening.
B, Examining the rectum. *C*, Examining the prostate.

any enlargement, irregularity
in shape, palpable mass,
tenderness, or softening (bogginess) (Fig. 20–2*C*).

8. Palpate the uterus and cervix in women.	Turn your finger to palpate the anterior rectal wall. Gently palpate the uterus and cervix. Note any enlargement, irregularity in shape, palpable mass, tenderness, or softening (bogginess).
9. Examine fecal material.	Withdraw your gloved finger and examine the fecal material on the glove for color (brown, gray, yellow, black) and consistency (watery, loose, greasy, formed, hard). Using a Hemoccult card (Fig. 20–3) test the stool for occult blood.

	Normal Findings	*Abnormal Findings*
Perianal tissue	No lesions, masses, erythema, or skin breakdown; tissue may appear slightly darker in pigmentation	Poor hygiene, erythema, ecchymosis, skin breakdown, decubitus ulcers, fistula openings, sinus tracts, abscesses, masses, or lesions
Anus	Appears slightly reddened and closed by voluntary sphincter; no lesions, masses, protrusions, hemorrhoids; patient may feel urge to defecate when finger is inserted; sphincter will normally tighten snuggly around finger.	Erythema, ecchymosis, edema, skin breakdown, decubitus ulcer, rectal prolapse (rosette), hemorrhoids, polyps, protrusions, lesions, masses, lacerations, fissures, fistulas, sinus tracts, and poor sphincter tone

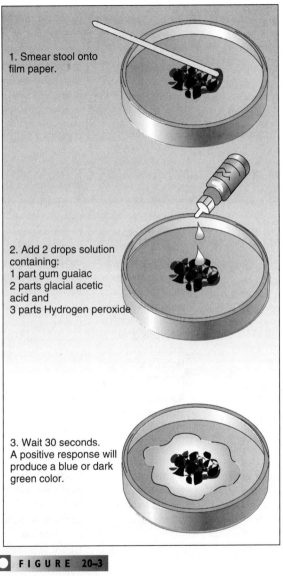

1. Smear stool onto film paper.

2. Add 2 drops solution containing:
1 part gum guaiac
2 parts glacial acetic acid and
3 parts Hydrogen peroxide

3. Wait 30 seconds. A positive response will produce a blue or dark green color.

FIGURE 20-3

Guaiac testing of stool.

Rectum	Smooth, without masses, lesions, tenderness	Tenderness, lesions, masses, or abnormalities; palpable rectal shelf (often secondary to peritoneal metastatic tissue); presence of a "high mass" descending against fingertip when the patient bears down
Prostate	Palpable only after onset of puberty; normally not >1 cm protruding into rectum; rubbery and smooth to palpation; two lateral lobes and median sulcus may be distinguishable; should be nontender, without palpable masses	Protrusion into rectum of >1 cm; enlarged, nodular, or irregular in shape; boggy or tender to palpation; any hard palpable mass
Uterus and cervix	Rubbery, smooth, and nontender	Any enlargement, irregularity of surface, palpable mass, or tenderness
Fecal material	Normally formed, brown stool, without frank or occult blood	Yellow, gray, or black stool; watery, loose, hard, or impacted stool; frank or occult blood (guaiac or Hemoccult test required)

Clinical Notes

Occasionally patients present with a foreign object in the rectum as their chief complaint. Digital examination should be done carefully so as not to push the object further down into the rectum.

If a Hemoccult test is positive, the patient should be referred for further testing to rule out colorectal malignancy.

Sexual assault or abuse must be considered whenever anal bruising or lacerations are observed.

Geriatric Considerations

	Normal Findings:
Rectum	Relaxation of the internal sphincter inhibited
Prostate	Enlarged

Clinical Notes

Difficulty starting and stopping the urine stream can be the result of an enlarged prostate. Obtain a clear picture of voiding patterns.

Pediatric Considerations

History

Stool pattern

Normal Findings	*Common Variations*	*Abnormal Findings*
Newborn		
Patent anus	Tight rectal sphincter	Meconium ileus
Passes meconium stool within 24 hours		Pencil-thin stools

21

Assessment of the Musculoskeletal System

HISTORY AND CURRENT STATUS QUESTIONS

Personal history

Arthritis, joint disease, collagen vascular disease, or cancer; illness affecting the strength or function of any muscle groups; recent or remote trauma (part of the body affected; resultant amputations, fractures, crushed, torn, or mangled muscles; orthopaedic or arthroscopic surgery); occupational or recreational activity likely to inflict a particular overuse injury

Family history

Family members with rheumatoid arthritis, gout, osteoarthritis, lupus, sickle cell

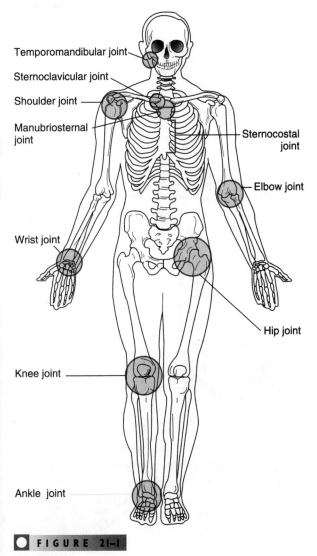

Temporomandibular joint

Sternoclavicular joint

Shoulder joint

Manubriosternal joint

Sternocostal joint

Elbow joint

Wrist joint

Hip joint

Knee joint

Ankle joint

FIGURE 21–1

Bones and joints.

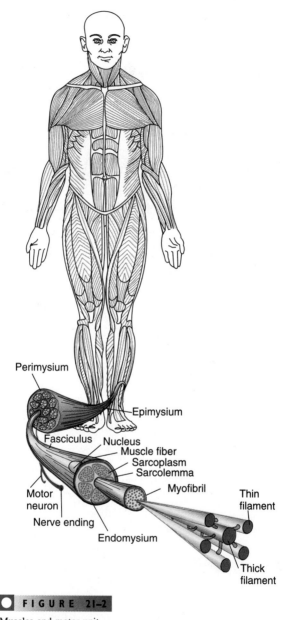

Perimysium

Epimysium

Fasciculus

Nucleus

Muscle fiber

Sarcoplasm

Sarcolemma

Myofibril

Thin filament

Motor neuron

Nerve ending

Endomysium

Thick filament

FIGURE 21–2

Muscles and motor unit.

TABLE 21–1
Classification of Joints

Type of Joint	Example	Description
Synarthrosis		*No movement is permitted*
Suture	Cranial sutures	United by thin layer of fibrous tissue
Synchondrosis	Joint between the epiphysis and diaphysis of long bones	A temporary joint in which the cartilage is replaced by bone later in life
Amphiarthrosis		Slightly *movable joint*
Symphysis	Symphysis pubis	Bones are connected by a fibrocartilage disk
Syndesmosis	Radius–ulna articulation	Bones are connected by ligaments
Diarthrosis (synovial)		*Freely movable*
		Enclosed by joint capsule, lined with synovial membrane
Ball and socket	Hip	Widest range of motion, movement in all planes
Hinge	Elbow	Motion limited to flexion and extension in a single plane
Pivot	Atlantoaxis	Motion limited to rotation
Condyloid	Wrist between radius and carpals	Motion in two planes at right angles to each other, but no radial rotation
Saddle	Thumb at carpometacarpal joint	Motion in two planes at right angles to each other, but no axial rotation
Gliding	Intervertebral	Motion limited to gliding

disease, congenital deformities of the bones or muscles, progressive myositis, multiple sclerosis, muscular dystrophy,

T A B L E   21–2
Muscle Function Terminology

Term	Definition and Example
Abduction	Lateral movement of a body part away from the midline of the body. *Example: The arm is abducted when it is moved away from the body.*
Adduction	Lateral movement of a body part toward the midline of the body. *Example: The arm is moved from an outstretched position to a position alongside the body.*
Circumduction	Movement of the distal part of the limb to trace a complete circle while the proximal end of the bone remains fixed. *Example: The leg is outstretched and moved in a circle.*
Flexion	The state of being bent.
Extension	The state of being in a straight line.
Hyperextension	The state of exaggerated extension. It often results in an angle >180 degrees. *Example: The spine is hyperextended when looking overhead, toward the ceiling.*
Dorsiflexion	Backward bending of the hand or foot. *Example: The foot is in dorsiflexion when the toes are brought up as though to point them at the knee.*
Plantar flexion	Flexion of the foot. *Example: The foot is in plantar flexion in the footdrop position.*
Rotation	Turning on an axis; the turning of a body part on the axis provided by its joint. *Example: A thumb is rotated when it is moved to make a circle.*
Internal rotation	A body part turning on its axis toward the midline of the body. *Example: A leg is rotated internally when it turns inward at the hip and the toes point toward the midline of the body.*
External rotation	A body part turning on its axis away from the midline of the body. *Example: A leg is rotated externally when it turns outward at the hip and the toes point away from the midline of the body.*

Table continued on following page

TABLE 21–2
Muscle Function Terminology *Continued*

Term	Definition and Example
Special Movements	
Pronation	The assumption of the prone position. *Example: Lying flat on the abdomen.*
Supination	The assumption of the supine position. *Example: Lying flat on the back*
Inversion	Movement of the sole of the foot inward (occurs at the ankle)
Eversion	Movement of the sole of the foot outward (occurs at the ankle)

	myasthenia gravis, polio, or cancer (relation of the family member to the patient, age of onset of the illness, and if the family member is deceased, illness or condition responsible for death)
Pain?	Provocative/palliative factors, quality, region (joint, muscle), severity, and timing (at rest, with exercise, a considerable time after exertion, upon awakening, or with extreme temperature or weather changes (PQRST; see Fig. 15–2)
Change in range of motion (ROM)?	Limited ability to move a particular joint, inability to bend at the waist, reach, grasp, hold, lift, stretch, walk, run, turn the head, sit, stand, or lie down as previously able

Change in size of an extremity or swelling of a joint?	Insidious or acute onset; associated edema, erythema, ecchymosis, pain, or heat of the affected area; trauma
Erythema?	Does the patient complain of erythema or areas of reddened skin surrounding a joint or extremity?
Temperature?	Fever (measured with a thermometer; oral or rectally), highest temperature recorded; joints, surrounding tissues, or extremities hot to the touch
Crepitus?	Unusual creaking or cracking sounds whenever a joint is moved or palpated
Deformity?	Malalignment, new or poorly healed fracture, arthritic nodule, tumor, or abnormal curvature (as in the spine)
Loss of height?	Osteoporosis in elderly (more often women) if unrelated to surgical procedures; severe kyphosis (hunched back) or compression fractures of the spine
Muscle weakness?	Muscles affected, characteristics (unilateral or bilateral, constant or intermittent, insidious or acute onset), associated with any trauma or surgery, effect on ADL

PHYSICAL EXAMINATION

Equipment

Tape measure
Goniometer

Procedures, Techniques, and Findings

1. Assess the patient's posture, stance, and gait.

   Observe the patient's posture, stance, and gait, inconspicuously as he/she enters the examining room.

2. Prepare the patient for the examination.

   Ask the patient to undress to his/her underwear. Instruct the patient to stand, sit, or lie down as necessary through the course of the examination.

3. Inspect for any gross abnormalities.

   Note any gross, or obvious abnormalities that are easily noticed on an initial glancing head to toe inspection (i.e., amputations, congenital deformities of extremities, contractures, paralysis, etc.).

4. Inspect and palpate the skin and surrounding tissue of all bones, joints and muscle groups to be examined.

   Refer to Chapter 6, Assessment of the Skin, Hair, and Nails.

5. Inspect and palpate the temporomandibular joint (TMJ) and jaw (Fig. 21–3).

   Inspect and palpate for abnormalities, deformities, masses, tenderness, or asymmetry. Place two or three fingertips of each hand over the TMJ joints simultaneously. Ask the patient to open widely and close the mouth two or three times. Palpate for any unusual clicking sounds, sliding, or "catching" of the joint. With the patient's mouth open as wide as possible, attempt to vertically insert three fingers held side by side between the upper and lower teeth. Ask the

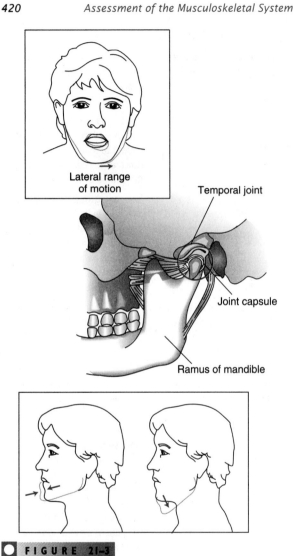

Lateral range of motion

Temporal joint

Joint capsule

Ramus of mandible

FIGURE 21-3

Range of motion: temporol mandibular joint and jaw.

patient to slide the lower jaw forward and from side to side, so that the lower teeth protrude beyond and over lap the upper teeth in each instance.

6. Inspect and palpate the neck and spine.

Inspect and palpate the neck and cervical spine. Then inspect and palpate the full length of the spine with the patient standing erect and again with the patient bending over at the waist. Observe the spinal curvature from directly behind the patient, and again from a side view. Normally the cervical spine is concave, the thoracic spine convex, and the lumbar spine concave. Note any abnormal curvatures of the spine, palpable masses, tenderness, or irregularities of alignment.

7. Assess the ROM of the neck (Fig. 21–4).

Flexion: touch chin to chest.

Hyperextension: bend head backward with chin pointing toward ceiling.

Rotation: turn head to the left and right with ears facing the back and chest.

Lateral bending: bend head laterally with ear toward shoulder.

8. Assess the ROM of the spine (Figure 21–5).

Flexion: bend forward at the waist.

Extension: bend backward at the waist.

Rotation: with feet planted and

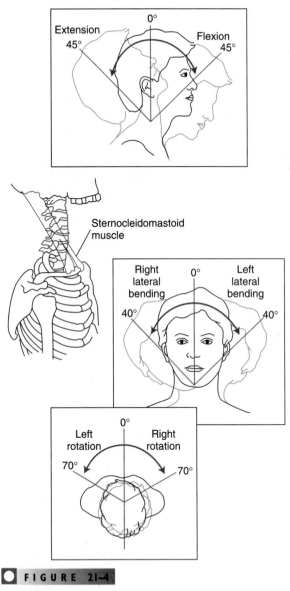

FIGURE 21-4

Range of motion: neck.

toes pointing forward, rotate the torso so that the shoulders attempt to face forward and backward.

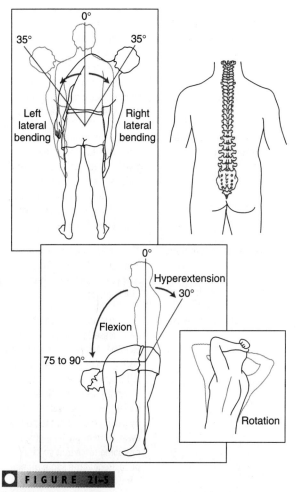

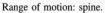

FIGURE 21-5

Range of motion: spine.

Lateral bending: bend laterally at the waist with shoulders toward feet.

9. Inspect and palpate the upper and lower extremities, assessing each joint and associated muscle groups for:

Work your way down from top to bottom, assessing first the right and then the left side. Begin with the shoulders. Assess the right and then the left shoulder, the right and then the left elbow, etc., moving down through the wrists, fingers, hips, knees, ankles, and toes.

Condition of skin and surrounding tissue

Inspect the skin and surrounding tissue for erythema, swelling, edema, masses, and lesions. Palpate for temperature, tenderness, crepitus (abnormal sounds), masses, or bony abnormalities.

Contralateral symmetry

Assess contralateral symmetry. Note any difference in size, shape, position, or alignment of like joints.

Muscle tone and strength

Muscle tone and strength may be assessed at the same time as ROM. Assess muscle tone by noting the degree of resistance felt on passive range of motion. Normally a slight resistance will be felt. Assess muscle strength by asking the patient to pull away from or push against an opposing force that you impose. Repeat the same maneuver with the contralateral joint

	and assess bilateral muscle strength.
Stability of joint	Assess the stability of each joint. In general, grasp and stabilize the joint on the proximal side with one hand while attempting to move the joint with the other hand from the distal end. Note any abnormal movements, crepitus, unusual sounds, abnormal ROM, or tenderness associated with these maneuvers. To further differentiate suspected tendon or ligament damage, refer to the special maneuvers described for each specific joint.
Range of motion	Put each joint through full passive range of motion (as detailed below). Note the angle at which the joint is freely able to bend in each position. Compare the ROM of contralateral joints. For greater accuracy measure the joint angles with a goniometer (Fig. 21–6).

10. Shoulders

Range of motion (Fig. 21–7)	Flexion: lift arm forward and above head with arm straight.
	Horizontal flexion: abduct arm straight and horizontal to the floor, then move arm backward toward the spine.
	Extension: move arm backward with arm straight.

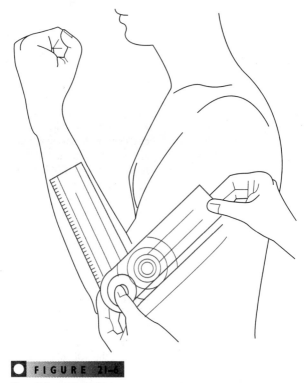

FIGURE 21-6

Use of the goniometer.

Horizontal extension: abduct arm horizontal to floor and then bring arm across chest.

Abduction: lift arm straight up above head.

Adduction: adduct arm toward midline of trunk.

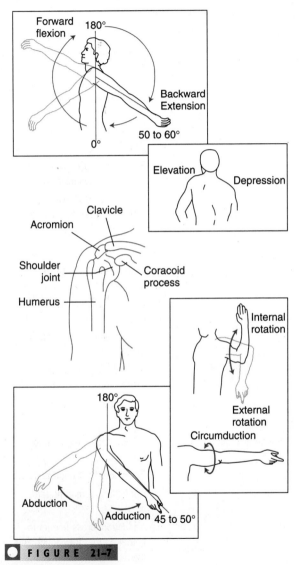

FIGURE 21–7

Range of motion: shoulders.

Special maneuvers

11. Elbows

Range of motion (Fig. 21–8)

Flexion: bend lower arm up toward biceps.

Extension: Open arm to resting fully extended position.

Hyperextension: extend arm beyond normal resting position.

Supination: turn lower arm so that front faces upward.

Pronation: turn lower arm so that front faces downward.

Special maneuvers

12. Wrists

Range of motion (Fig. 21–9)

Flexion: flex wrist toward lower arm.

Extension: extend wrist backward.

Radial deviation: deviate wrist toward radius.

Ulnar deviation: deviate wrist toward ulna.

Special maneuvers

13. Fingers

Range of motion (Fig. 21–10)

Flexion: close fingers into a fist.

Extension: fully open fingers.

Abduction: spread fingers apart.

Adduction: cross fingers together so that they touch and overlap.

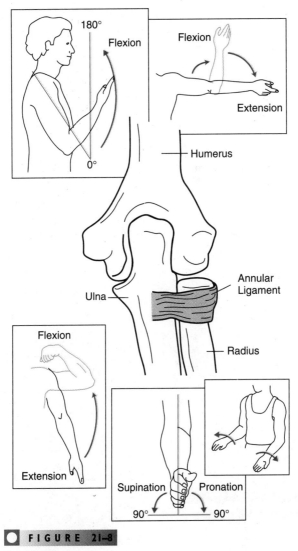

FIGURE 21–8

Range of motion: elbows.

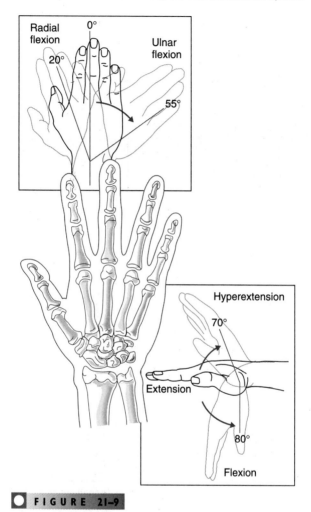

⬤ FIGURE 21–9

Range of motion: wrists.

Opposition: touch each finger
with the thumb of the same
hand.

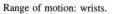

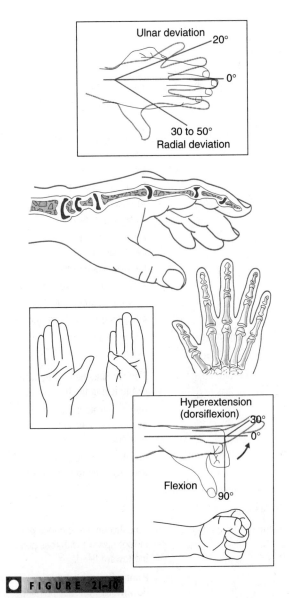

Ulnar deviation
20°
0°
30 to 50°
Radial deviation

Hyperextension
(dorsiflexion)
30°
0°
Flexion
90°

FIGURE 21-10

Range of motion: fingers.

Special maneuvers

14. Hips

Range of motion (Fig. 21–11)

Flexion with straight knee: raise leg straight up without bending the knee.

Flexion with knee bent: raise leg straight up with knee bent.

Extension: lie prone and extend leg backward.

Abduction: abduct partially flexed leg outward.

Adduction: adduct partially flexed leg inward.

Internal rotation: flex knee and swing foot away from midline.

External rotation: flex knee and swing foot toward midline.

Special maneuvers

15. Knees

Range of motion (Fig. 21–12)

Flexion: Fully bend knee with calf touching thigh.

Hyperextension: extend knee beyond normal point of extension.

Internal rotation: rotate knee and lower leg toward midline.

Special maneuvers

16. Ankles

Range of motion (Fig. 21–13)

Dorsiflexion: bend dorsal part of foot upward with toes pointing toward head.

Plantar flexion: bend foot downward with toes pointing downward.

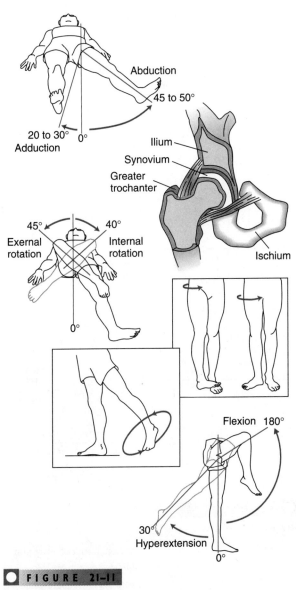

Abduction
45 to 50°

20 to 30°
Adduction
0°

Ilium
Synovium
Greater
trochanter

Ischium

45°
Exernal
rotation

40°
Internal
rotation

0°

Flexion 180°

30°
Hyperextension
0°

FIGURE 21-11

Range of motion: hips.

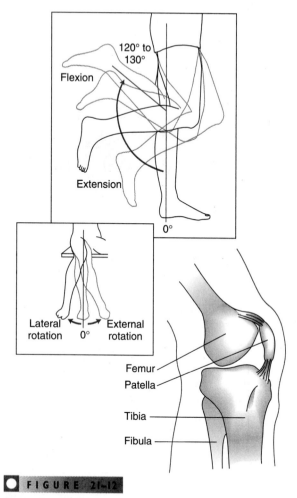

FIGURE 21-12

Range of motion: knees.

Eversion: turn foot away from midline.

Inversion: turn foot toward midline.

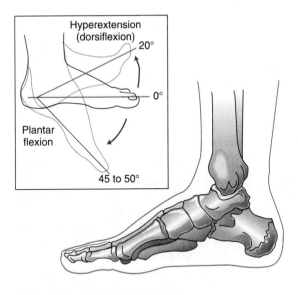

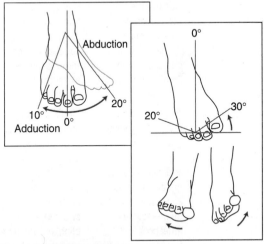

Range of motion: ankles.

Special maneuvers

17. Toes

Range of motion (Fig. 21–14)

Flexion: curl toes under foot.

Extension: lift toes to point upward.

Abduction: spread toes apart.

Adduction: normally unable.

Special maneuvers

	Normal Findings	*Abnormal Findings*
Posture	Ability to stand erect, with head up, face forward, arms hanging straight at the sides, shoulders and hips parallel, legs straight with both knees and feet side by side and a few inches apart; contralateral extremities equal in size, shape, and length, and symmetrical	Inability to stand erect, exhibiting hunched, bent, stooped posture; abnormal curvature of the spine, as in kyphosis (accentuated lordosis) or scoliosis (lateral bending of the spine) (Fig. 21–15); contractures or deformities of the extremities
Stance	Ability to stand comfortably without assistance or extrinsic support and without swaying or loss of balance on both feet or on one foot at a time; both feet firmly planted a few inches apart with toes and heels on	Inability to stand either on two feet or on one foot without assistance or support; evidence of uneven distribution of weight: swaying, stumbling, or loss of balance, favoring one foot, standing on the heels, toes, or

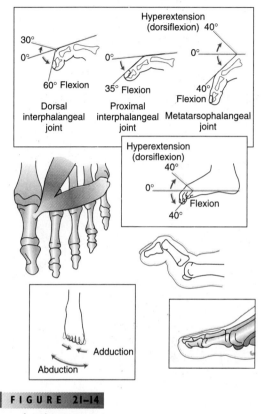

Range of motion: toes.

the ground; toes
pointing forward
and the weight
evenly distributed
on both feet

edges of the feet,
uneven depths of
footprints, etc.; toes
pointing either lat-
erally or medially

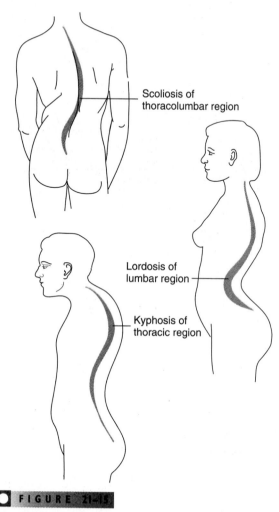

Scoliosis of thoracolumbar region

Lordosis of lumbar region

Kyphosis of thoracic region

○ **FIGURE 21–15**

Abnormalities of the spine.

| Gait | Ability to walk with equal and symmet- | rather than straight ahead
Evidence of an un-steady gait, exces- |

	rical strides with respect to timing, weight bearing, and distance; steps consisting of a rhythmic planting of first the heel and then the toe of the foot; toes consistently pointing forward; slight swaying back and forth while walking, but no unsteadiness or loss of balance	sive swaying, loss of balance, shuffling, limping, propulsive, veering in one direction, exhibiting foot drop or foot lag or any irregularity in the timing of the stride
Skin		
Color	Slightly darker in areas most often exposed to sunlight and lighter in areas usually clothed (refer to Chapter 6, Assessment of the Skin, Hair, and Nails)	Hyper or hypopigmentation, erythema, ecchymosis, pale, ashen, gray, or cyanotic; redness suggests gouty arthritis, septic arthritis, or rheumatic fever
Lesions	No lesions, masses, lacerations, scars	Presence of macules, papules, vesicles, ulcers, lacerations, scars, masses, or other lesions; subcutaneous nodules may be present in rheumatoid arthritis and rheumatic fever
Swelling or edema	No swelling or edema	Swelling, edema (pitting or nonpitting) (see Fig. 16–5) or palpable effusion

		of an underlying joint
Skinfolds	Symmetrical in number and size over contralateral extremities	Asymmetry of contralateral skinfolds may suggest malalignment of a bone or joint (fracture or dislocation)
Temperature	Warm, not hot to touch	Hot to touch, tactile fever; "hot joint" may represent gouty arthritis, septic arthritis, rheumatic fever, cellulitis, or a localized infection in the skin or subcutaneous tissue
Muscles		
Contralateral symmetry	Contralateral muscle groups symmetrical in size, shape, contour, and position; tone and strength may vary normally, with increased tone and strength demonstrated on the dominant side	Asymmetry in size, shape, contour, diameter, position; Wide variance in tone or strength between contralateral muscle groups
Tone	A particular muscle or muscle group will have normal tone if slight resistance is demonstrated against passive ROM	Hypertonic muscle exhibits increased resistance to passive ROM; hypotonic muscle presents as boggy, fat, flabby or flaccid muscle that

		offers little or no resistance against passive ROM
Strength	Capable of providing significant resistance to the opposing force imposed; this resistance (or strength) should be relatively equal when compared to the contralateral muscle or muscle group; dominant hand and arm may normally be slightly stronger; normal muscle strength should range between 3 and 5, as described in Bates' assessment of muscle strength scale (Table 21–3)	Measure the size and circumference of any muscle or muscle groups that demonstrate weakness (or range from 0 to 2 on Bates' scale); smaller circumference and size of a particular muscle or muscle group may indicate atrophy; conversely, an unusually large muscle may indicate hypertrophy

T A B L E   21–3
Scale for Muscle Strength

Scale	
0	No muscular contraction
1	Barely flicker of contraction
2	Active movement with gravity removed
3	Active movement against gravity
4	Active movement against gravity and some resistance
5	Active movement against full resistance with no fatigue

Normal strength ranges from 3 to 5.

Adapted from Bates B: A Guide to Physical Examination and History Taking, 5th ed., p. 526. Philadelphia: JB Lippincott, 1991.

Bones and joints

Contralateral symmetry	Contralateral bones and joints should be symmetrical in size, shape, position, alignment, stability, and ROM	Asymmetry secondary to congenital abnormalities, arthritis, bony tumor, fractures, dislocations, adhesions, or surgery
Change in size or shape	Contralateral bones and joints equal in size and shape	
Position and alignment	Normally positioned and well aligned	Malalignment secondary to fracture, dislocation, congenital anomalies, or surgical procedures
Stability	No abnormal movements, ROM, or sounds upon movement of joints or use of special maneuvers	Instability of a joint without associated dislocation usually indicates tendon or ligament damage
ROM	Ability to move joints passively in all directions and degrees usual for the specific joints, as further described below	Inability or limited ability of a joint to passively move through ROM maneuvers because of stiffness or pain
Jaw (TMJ)	Ability to open and close the jaw freely without pain, clicking, or abnormal sounds, to admit three fingers held	Abnormal clicking sound when opening and closing the jaw; malalignment of the upper and

together and perpendicular to upper and lower teeth, and to move lower jaw forward so that the bottom teeth overlap the top teeth, and side to side so that the bottom side teeth overlap the top side teeth

lower jaw; inability to move lower jaw sideways or forward; lockjaw (inability to open or close mouth); pain on mastication or movement of the jaw

Neck

Concave curvature of the neck or cervical spine when viewed from the side; no palpable pain or masses

Normal ROM

Flexion: 70 to 90 degrees

Hyperextension: 55 degrees

Rotation: 70 degrees

Lateral bending: 35 degrees

Pain, palpable masses, compression fractures, lesions, masses, or abnormal curvature; tight palpable cordlike trapezius muscle suggests muscle spasm; chronic pain may be secondary to postural strain; acute recurrent neck pain may be secondary to a herniated intervertebral disc pressing on a nerve root, or cervical spondylosis (degenerative joint disease of one or more discs in the cervical spine with narrowing of the disc spaces and presence of bony spurs)

Spine	Convex thoracic spine and concave lumbar sacral spine when viewed from the side; no abnormal lateral curvatures; no palpable masses, pain, compression fractures	Abnormal curvature of the spine, including kyphosis (an accentuated posterior curvature of the thoracic spine, lordosis), sway-back (an accentuated lumbar curvature), scoliosis (a lateral curvature of the spine), and ankylosing spondylitis (evidenced by the persistence of the lumbar concavity and failure of the spinous processes to separate when the patient bends over at the waist); a herniated disc may be tender on palpation; spondylolisthesis (a forward slipping and fusing of the vertebra) may be palpable
	Normal ROM	
	Flexion: 75 degrees	
	Extension: 30 degrees	
	Rotation: 30 degrees	
	Lateral bending: 35 degrees	
Shoulder	Ability to move freely on passive range of motion; no swelling, ecchymosis, lesions, or tenderness; no fractures or dislocation; shoulders symmetrical in size, shape,	Pain secondary to arthritis, inflammation, infection, bursitis, tendonitis, bony spurs, calcific deposits, masses, fractures, or dislocations; frozen shoulder (in-

contour, muscle tone and strength, and ROM

Normal ROM:

Flexion:
180 degrees

Horizontal flexion:
130 degrees

Extension:
60 degrees

Horizontal extension:
45 degrees

Abduction:
180 degrees

Adduction:
45 degrees

ability to abduct the arm without characteristic "shrugging") suggests a rupture of the supraspinatous tendon or rotator cuff injury

Elbow

Normal ROM:

Flexion:
150 degrees

Extension:
150 degrees

Hyperextension:
0 to 10 degrees

Supination:
90 degrees

Pronation:
90 degrees

Subcutaneous nodules on the extensor surface of the ulna suggest rheumatoid arthritis; a tender lateral epicondyle suggests tennis elbow; swelling, inflammation, or thickening of the olecranon gooves suggests olecranon arthritis or bursitis

Wrist

Normal ROM:

Flexion: 80 to 90 degrees

Extension:
70 degrees

Ganglion cyst (a cystic round, non-tender swelling along the tendon sheaths or joint

Radial deviation: 20 degrees

Ulnar deviation: 30 to 50 degrees

capsules on the dorsum of the hand or wrists that becomes more prominent when the wrist is flexed and obscured when the wrist is extended), carpal tunnel syndrome (compression of the median nerve that produces numbness and tingling over the palmar surface of the thumb, index, middle, and part of the ring finger, gonococcal arthritis: (unilateral tenderness of wrist; may be hot and erythematous)

Fingers

Normal ROM:

Flexion: 80 to 100 degrees (depends on specific joint)

Extension: 0 to 45 degrees (depending on specific joint)

Abduction: 20 degrees

Adduction: able to cross fingers together so that

Arthritic nodules and deformities; atrophy of the thenar eminence may indicate median nerve damage; atrophy of the hypothenar space may indicate ulnar nerve damage; felon (infection of a fingertip with infection in an adjacent fascial space); ten-

they touch and overlap

Opposition: able to touch each finger with the thumb of the same hand

don sheath infections (tenderness and swelling along the tendon sheath and partial flexion of the affected finger)

Dupuytren's contracture: progressive permanent thickening and contracture of the tendon sheath with resulting fixed flexion of the affected finger and a palpable hard cordlike tendon sheath

Degenerative joint disease: hard painless nodules on the dorsolateral aspects of interphalangeal joints; radial deviation of the distal phalanx; Heberden's nodes on the distal interphalangeal (DIP) joints; Bouchard's nodes on the proximal interphalangeal (PIP) joints; sparing of the metacarpophalangeal (MCP) joints

Gout: asymmetrical involvement of the

joints; a knobby swelling that may be hot and painful and may ulcerate and discharge chalky urates; uric acid usually high

Acute rheumatoid arthritis: symmetrical involvement of the joints; tenderness, stiffness; nodules and deformities of the wrist, MCP, and PIP joints with sparing of the DIP joints

Chronic rheumatoid arthritis: chronic swelling and thickening of the MCP and PIP joints; interosseous muscular atrophy of the hand; ulnar deviation of the fingers; nodules, swan neck and boutonnière deformities of the fingers

Hips	Normal ROM:	
	Flexion with straight knee: 90 degrees	Arthritis evidenced by pain and limited ROM of the hip
	Flexion with knee bent: 110 to 120 degrees	Flexion deformity of the hip: test by flexing the knee

Extension:
30 degrees

Abduction: 45 to 50
degrees

Adduction: 20 to 30
degrees

Internal rotation: 35
to 40 degrees

External rotation:
45 degrees

on one side and
watching for involuntary flexing of
the opposite side

Pelvic tilt: unequal
height of the ileac
crests may be secondary to unequal
lengths of the legs
or adduction/abduction deformities
of the hip

Aseptic necrosis
of the hip: secondary to sickle cell
disease

Sacroiliac pain: test
by having supine
patient firmly flex
the opposite knee
against the abdomen while hyperextending the other
extended leg by
dangling it off the
edge of the examining table

Knees	Normal ROM:	
	Flexion: 130 degrees	Bow knees (genu varum), knock knees (genu valgum), Flexion contracture (inability to extend joint fully), bony enlargement (degenerative joint disease)
	Hyperextension: 15 degrees	
	Internal rotation: 10 degrees	

Tenosynovitis: loss of hollows above and adjacent to patella suggests synovial thickening

Ballottement of patella suggests synovial thickening or fluid; positive bulge sign (milk upward on the medial side of patella, then tap the lateral side of the patella and watch for returning bulge of fluid)

Thickening, bogginess, or tenderness suggests synovial inflammation of the knee

Instability

Abduction mobility: relaxation or tear of the medial collateral ligament

Adduction mobility: relaxation or tear of the lateral collateral ligament

Anterior mobility: anterior cruciate ligament damage

		Posterior mobility: posterior cruciate ligament damage
		Torn medial or lateral meniscus
Ankles	Normal ROM:	
	Dorsiflexion: 20 degrees	Pain, swelling, erythema, or stiffness; arthritis may be difficult to differentiate from edema or cellulitis
	Plantar flexion: 45 degrees	
	Eversion: 20 degrees	
	Inversion: 30 degrees	
Toes	Normal ROM:	
	Flexion: 35 to 60 degrees (depending on the specific joint)	Rheumatoid nodules; tenderness in the small metatarsophalangeal (MTP) joints is an early sign of rheumatoid arthritis; pain or swelling of the first MTP joint of the great toe suggests gout
	Extension: 0 to 90 degrees (depending on specific joint)	
	Abduction: varies	
	Adduction: normally unable	
		Halux valgus: great toe abnormally abducted with medial deviation
		Bunion: usually a painful swelling of

the MTP joint of
the great toe

Flat feet: absence
of normal arch
of the sole of the
foot; the sole lies
flat on the floor

Clinical Notes

Be gentle when examining the patient, and take care not to
inflict harm by expecting the patient to do more than he
or she is capable of. Never force a joint beyond its
natural limit while guiding it through passive range of
motion or special maneuvers.

In many conditions, the use of imaging modalities such as
roentgenography, myelography, or bone scanning may be
necessary to confirm suspected diagnosis.

Geriatric Considerations

	Normal Findings
Muscles	Decline in mass, tone, and strength
Bones and joints	Narrowing of joint spaces due to a thinning of cartilage; bony prominences of the vertebrae and ribs
	Iliac crest sharpened as a result of a loss of subcutaneous fat; diminished mobility, flexibility, and range of motion

Clinical Notes

Common arthritic changes of the wrist and knees result in
joint enlargement, crepitus, stiffness, and pain.

Shrinking and stiffening of ligaments and tendons and narrowing of joint spaces can limit range of motion. Slowly
and gently assess movement of joints to limit pain and
potential injury.

Pediatric Considerations

History

Birth injuries?
History of congenital hip dysplasia in extended family?
Sports?
Trauma?

Normal Findings	Common Variations	Abnormal Findings
Newborn		Postdelivery clavicular fracture
	Adduction of the forefoot, may be manipulated to neutral or an overcorrected position	Metatarsus adductus: rigid adduction of forefoot
Equal gluteal folds		Congenital hip dysplasia: positive Ortolani sign ("click" heard when hips are flexed and abducted to examining table) and/or limited abduction
Infant		
Bowing of legs, which begins to disappear at 18 months to 2 years		
Fat pad under arch of foot, "flatfooted" appearance		
Child and Adolescent		
Wide-based gait with some pronation of feet until age 2 years		Scoliosis: "S" curve of spine; asymmetry of shoulders and hips

Increased lumbar curvature in the toddler, resulting in a protuberant abdomen

Knock-kneed appearance in the preschool child and early school-age child

>3 inches between ankles when knees are together

22

Assessment of the Nervous System

HISTORY AND CURRENT STATUS QUESTIONS

Headache?

Location; unilateral or bilateral; character and severity of pain; acute or gradual onset; pattern of occurrence—constant or chronic recurrent, worsening over time or stable in intensity, time of onset, duration, precipitating or associated factors such as particular activities, time of day, or stressful events, effect of movement such as change in head position, coughing or sneezing; associated symptoms such as nausea and vomiting, nasal congestion, fever, relief measures tried and their effectiveness.

Injury?

Description, including any loss of consciousness and its duration; date of occurrence; precipitating or prodromal events such as faintness or pain, treatment; residual effects.

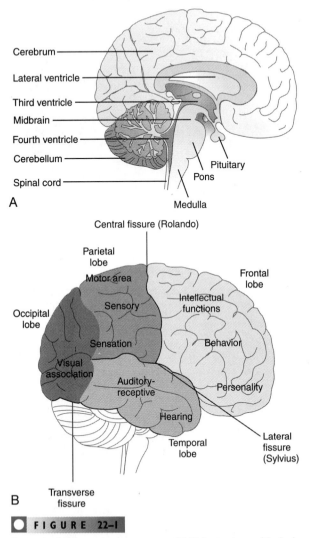

FIGURE 22–1

Anatomy of the central nervous system. *(A)* Main structures of the brain. *(B)* Lobes of the cerebral hemispheres and their specialized functions.

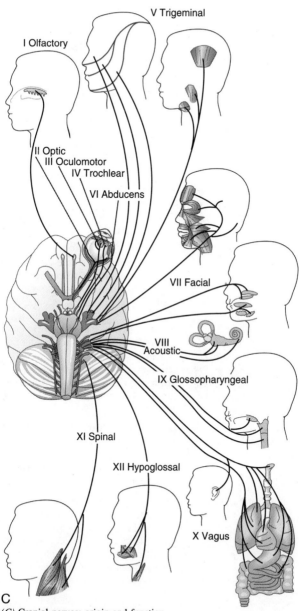

I Olfactory

V Trigeminal

II Optic
III Oculomotor
IV Trochlear
VI Abducens

VII Facial

VIII Acoustic

IX Glossopharyngeal

XI Spinal

XII Hypoglossal

X Vagus

C

(C) Cranial nerves: origin and function.

Dizziness/light-headedness?	Frequency; duration; time of occurrence; precipitating factors, such as change in position, or specific activities.
Fainting?	Frequency; duration; time of occurrence; precipitating factors; position at time of occurrence; warning signs; appearance before and after syncope; feeling after return of consciousness.
Vertigo (sense you or the room about you is spinning)?	Time and type (sudden or gradual) of onset; severity; constant or intermittent; associated symptoms (nausea, vomiting, ataxia); precipitating factors; type and effectiveness of relief measures used.
Seizures?	Type; sequence of seizure effects on the body, duration; postictal reaction (e.g., sleep, confusion, weakness, headache) and its duration; aura; age at onset; cause if known; frequency, any recent change in frequency; time of last seizure; exacerbating factors (e.g., stress, fatigue, specific activities, omission of medication); treatment; side effects of medication; pattern of compliance with treatment regimen.
Tremors or other involuntary movements?	Date and type of onset; body part(s) affected; exacerbating factors (e.g., purposeful activity, rest, anxiety); ameliorating factors (e.g., rest, activity, alcohol).
Paresis or paralysis?	Date and type of onset; body parts affected; generalized or localized; unilateral or bilateral; type of progression, if any; effect of rest; effect of repeated activity; other exacerbating or ameliorating factors; associated symptoms.

Coordination problems?	Loss of balance when walking; history of falls; clumsy movements; listing to one side; date and type of onset; associated symptoms; exacerbating factors; ameliorating factors.
Paresthesias? (Loss of sensation)	Date and type of onset; type (e.g., tingling, pins and needles); area of body affected; constant or intermittent; effect on daily activities; exacerbating factors; ameliorating factors.
Difficulty speaking?	Type (e.g., difficulty forming words, saying what is meant); date and type of onset; constant or intermittent; exacerbating factors; ameliorating factors; associated symptoms.
Difficulty swallowing?	Solids and/or liquids; drooling; type and time of onset; constant or intermittent; exacerbating factors; ameliorating factors; associated symptoms.
History of nervous system disease?	Type of disorder (e.g., stroke, spinal cord injury, meningitis, encephalitis); date of occurrence; treatment; residual effects.
Medications? (OTC and prescription)	Name; dose; route; frequency; reason for use.
Use of alcohol?	Type; amount (glasses, bottles, pint, half pint); frequency (e.g., daily, two to three times per week, two to three times per month); pattern of use (weekends only, when out or with company, with dinner, evenings, morning); type and frequency of any "hangover" symptoms; occurrence of blackout periods.
Drug abuse?	Type of drug(s) used; route; amount; frequency; length of time used;

effects; date and type of any treatment.

Exposure to environmental or occupational hazards?

Type of hazard; type and duration of exposure.

PHYSICAL EXAMINATION

Equipment

Cotton; flashlight; newspaper (or other printed material); ophthalmoscope; otoscope; reflex hammer; sterile needle; Snellen chart; tape measure; tongue depressor; tuning fork; various objects of different shapes (key, marble, coin); vials (stoppered) containing peppermint, coffee, or other familiar aromatic substance, salt or vinegar, and hot and cold water.

Procedures, Techniques, and Findings

Procedure	Technique
Assess mental status	See Chapter 4.
Assess speech and language function	
Expressive component of speech	Ask patient to repeat one or two phrases. Note clarity, fluency and ability to repeat the phrases without hesitancy or substitution.
	Show the patient five different objects and ask him or her to name each.
Receptive component of speech	Ask the patient to follow a simple one-step command such as "Close your eyes."
Assess cranial nerve (Table 22–1) function	
CN I (olfactory nerve)	Ask the patient to close his or her eyes.

Functions of the Cranial Nerves

Cranial Nerve		Sensory Function	Motor Function
I	Olfactory	Smell	
II	Optic	Sight	
III	Oculomotor		Extraocular eye movements, elevation of lids, pupillary constriction, control of lens shape
IV	Trochlear		Downward and inward eye movement
V	Trigeminal	Sensation of face, scalp, oral and nasal mucous membranes and the cornea	Chewing movements of the jaw
VI	Abducens		Lateral eye movement
VII	Facial	Taste on the anterior 2/3 of the tongue	Facial movement, eye closure, labial speech
VIII	Acoustic	Hearing and balance	
IX	Glosso-pharyngeal	Taste on the posterior third of the tongue, pharyngeal gag reflex, sensation from the ear drum and ear canal	Swallowing and phonation muscles of the pharynx
X	Vagus	Sensation from pharynx, viscera, carotid body, carotid sinus	Swallowing and talking muscles of the palate, pharynx, larynx
XI	Spinal		Trapezius and sternocleidomastoid muscle movement
XII	Hypoglossal		Tongue movement

Occlude one of the patient's nostrils.

Hold a familiar aromatic substance such as coffee, vanilla,

peppermint, or tobacco under the nonoccluded nostril.

Ask the patient to sniff and identify the odor.

Repeat for the other nostril.

Note unilateral or bilateral decrease or loss of smell.

Repeat with a different familiar aromatic substance to determine if the patient can distinguish a difference between odors.

Test only when patient complains of loss of smell or when assessing for an intracranial lesion.

CN II (optic nerve)

Test visual acuity and visual fields (see Chapter 7).

Examine the retina with an ophthalmoscope (see Chapter 7).

CN III, IV, and VI (oculomotor, trochlear, and abducens nerves)

Check pupils for size, regularity, equality, reaction to light, and accommodation.

Test extraocular movements by having the patient follow your finger as you move it through the six cardinal positions of gaze. Note limited or abnormal movement (see Chapter 7).

CN V (trigeminal nerve)

Motor function

Ask the patient to clench the teeth.

Palpate the temporal and masseter muscles (Fig. 22–2)

and push down on the chin to try and separate the jaws while the teeth are clenched (see Fig. 7–3).

Note decreased strength or asymmetric jaw movement.

Sensory function

Check light touch sensation in all three sensory divisions of the trigeminal nerve:

Ophthalmic

Maxillary

Ask the patient to close his or her eyes.

Proceed to alternately touch a cotton wisp or sterile pin to the patient's right forehead, cheek, and chin.

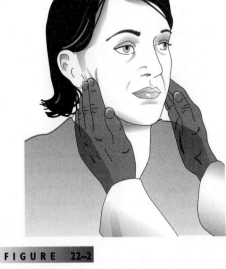

● FIGURE 22–2

Palpation of the masseter muscles to check motor function of CN V (trigeminal nerve).

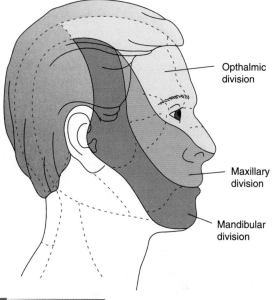

Opthalmic division

Maxillary division

Mandibular division

⬤ FIGURE 22–3

Sensory divisions of CN V (trigeminal nerve).

Mandibular (Fig. 22–3)	Ask patient to identify what is felt and where.
	Repeat for the left side.
	Note absent, decreased or un-equal sensation.
Check the corneal reflex (also tests motor function of CN VII)	Ask patient to remove contact lenses, if worn.
	Direct patient to look straight ahead.
	Bring a wisp of cotton in from the side and lightly touch the cornea (not just the conjunc-

tiva) of each eye in turn (Fig. 22–4).

Observe for bilateral blinking.

Omit in a routine screening examination.

CN VII (facial nerve)
  Sensory function
    Test taste

Touch the anterior tongue on both sides with a cotton applicator that has been dipped in a sugar, salt, or lemon solution.

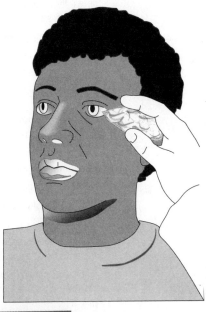

● FIGURE 22–4

Checking the corneal reflex.

	Ask the patient to identify the taste.
	Omit in a routine screening examination.
Motor function	Ask the patient to smile, frown, raise the eyebrows, show upper and lower teeth, keep eyes tightly closed as you try to open them (see Fig. 7–2), and puff out the cheeks.
	Observe for mobility and symmetry as these actions are performed.
	Press puffed cheeks in and note if air escapes equally from both sides.
CN VIII (acoustic nerve)	Test hearing (see Chapter 8).
CN IX and X (glossopharyngeal) and vagus nerves)	Ask patient to open the mouth and say "ah" as you depress the tongue with a tongue blade.
	Note movement of the uvula, soft palate, and tonsillar pillars.
	Touch the tongue blade to the posterior pharyngeal wall.
	Observe for gagging.
	Note quality of patient's voice.
CN XI (spinal accessory nerve)	Inspect the right and left sternocleidomastoid and trapezius muscles for equal size.
	Place your hand against the side of the patient's chin and face (Fig. 22–5A).
	Ask patient to turn head against this resistance.

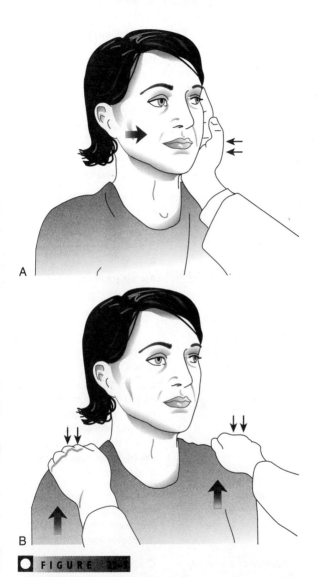

FIGURE

Checking function of CN XI (spinal accessory nerve) *(A)* by asking the patient to turn the head against the resistance of the examiner's hand placed on the side of the face and chin; *(B)* by having the patient shrug shoulders against the resistance of the examiner's hands.

Repeat for the opposite side.

Place your hands on the patient's shoulders.

Direct patient to shrug shoulders against the resistance of your hands (Fig. 22–5*B*).

Compare movement on right and left sides for equality.

CN XII (hypoglossal nerve)

Direct the patient to stick out the tongue.

Observe direction of protrusion and note any movement or wasting.

Ask patient to say "late date night."

Assess motor function (see Chapter 20)

Muscle mass and size

Ask patient to lie down and relax.

Inspect and palpate each muscle group, comparing muscles on the right side of the body with counterparts on the left side. Verify any perceived differences in size with a tape measure.

Muscle tone

Passively move each extremity through a full range of motion, noting any hypotonia or hypertonia (see Chapter 20).

Movement

Check voluntary and involuntary movement and range of motion (see Chapter 20).

Muscle strength

Ask patient to move each

T A B L E   22–2
Grading Scale for Motor Strength

Grade	Description
5/5	Normal muscle strength (i.e., full range of motion against examiner resistance)
4/5	Full range of motion of muscle that can be overcome with increased examiner resistance
3/5	Full range of motion of muscle against gravity only; is overcome with slight examiner resistance
2/5	Weak movement of muscle but insufficient to overcome gravity
1/5	Slight visible or palpable contraction muscle noted but no movement results
0/5	Complete paralysis

muscle group against your resistance (see Chapter 20).

Compare left side to right side and note symmetry and equality of strength.

Grade motor strength against gravity and resistance on a scale of 0 to 5, with 5 being normal and 0 complete paralysis (Table 22–2).

Gait

Observe the patient walk 10 to 20 feet away from you, turn, and return.

Note posture, rhythm, effort, symmetry of gait, and coordination of arm movement and arm swing.

Ask patient to walk heel to toe (tandem walk) along a straight line (Figure 22–6).

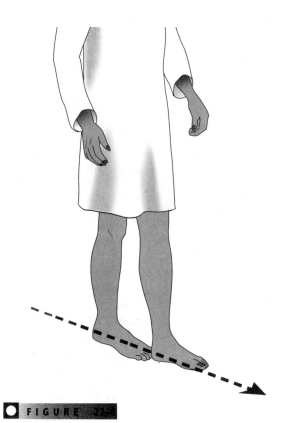

FIGURE 27-1

Tandem walk.

Assess balance and coor-
dination

Romberg's test

Have patient stand with feet
together and arms at sides.

Direct patient to close eyes
and maintain the position.

Wait 20 seconds and then tell
the patient to open the eyes
and relax.

Be prepared to catch the patient during this test if he or she should start to fall.

Arm drift test (Pronator drift)

Ask patient to put both arms straight out in front of the body with palms up, close the eyes, and hold this arm position for 10 to 15 seconds. Watch for any downward drift of the arms or pronation of the hands (Fig. 22–7).

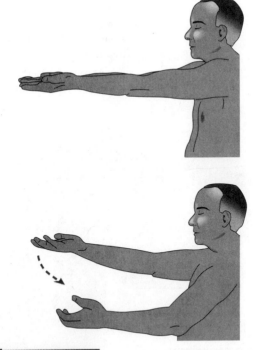

⬤ **FIGURE 22–7**

Arm drift (pronator drift) test.

Rapid alternating movement (RAM) test	Ask the patient to touch the right thumb to each finger of the right hand, going from index finger to little finger and back to the index finger.

Have patient repeat the action using the left hand.

OR

Ask patient to place the palms of the hands on the knees; lift the hands; turn them over; and touch the knees with the back of the hands.

Direct the patient to repeat this action as rapidly as possible (Fig. 22–8).

Finger-to-finger test	Ask the patient to touch your index finger and then his or

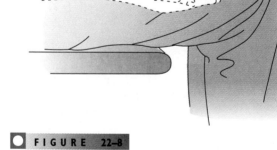

⬤ FIGURE 22–8

RAM test.

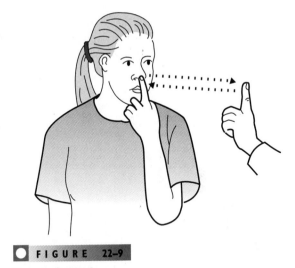

Finger-to-finger test.

	her own nose with his or her right and then left index finger (Fig. 22–9).
Finger-to-nose test	Ask patient to extend arms in front of him- or herself, close his or her eyes and touch the tip of the nose with the right and then the left index finger (Fig. 22–10).
	Direct the patient to continue to perform this alternating motion as quickly as possible.
Heel-to-shin test	Have the patient assume a dorsal recumbent position.
	Direct the patient to place the heel of the right foot just below the knee on the left shin

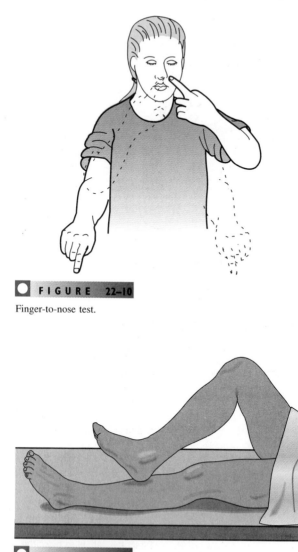

FIGURE 22-10

Finger-to-nose test.

FIGURE 22-11

Heel-to-shin test.

and run the heel down the shin to the ankle (Fig. 22–11).

Have the patient repeat the procedure with the left heel on the right shin.

Assess sensory function

Light touch

Ask patient to close eyes then stroke an area of the patient's skin with a wisp of cotton.

Ask the patient to identify the area touched and to describe the feeling.

Repeat on the opposite side of the body and compare results.

Repeat this procedure in a systematic manner, testing the hands, forearms, upper arms, torso, thigh, lower leg, and foot.

Superficial pain sensation

Ask patient to close eyes.

Gently touch the point of a sterile needle against the skin.

Randomly intersperse touches with the blunt end of the needle.

Allow at least 2 seconds between each touch.

Ask patient to indicate if sharpness or dullness is felt.

Progress in a systematic fashion as for light touch.

Dispose of used needle in a sharps container.

Temperature sensitivity

Ask patient to close eyes.

Touch a stoppered vial of hot

water to the patient's abdomen for 1 second, then touch a vial of cold water to the abdomen for 1 second.

Ask the patient to state which was hot and cold.

Repeat for the extremities.

Position sense

Ask patient to close eyes.

Move the fingers and toes up or down, one by one.

Ask the patient to state in which direction the digit has been moved (Fig. 22–12).

Check three or four digits on each hand and foot.

Vibration sense

Ask patient to close eyes.

Tap the tines of a tuning fork on the heel of your hand to set it vibrating.

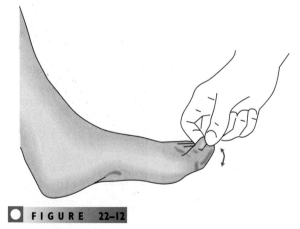

FIGURE 22–12

Testing position sense.

Place it firmly over the distal interphalangeal joint of the patient's finger.

Ask the patient what he or she feels.

Repeat for the distal joint of the patient's great toe.

Test more proximal bony prominences if vibration sense is impaired.

Stereognosis

Ask the patient to close his or her eyes.

Place a familiar object, such as a key, in the patient's hands (Fig. 22–13).

Ask the patient to name it.

Repeat for the other hand using a different familiar object, such as a coin.

Graphesthesia

Ask the patient to close his or her eyes.

Trace a single number or letter on the palm of the patient's hand with a blunt object, such as the cap of a pen (Fig. 22–14).

Ask the patient to identify what was traced.

Repeat for the other hand using different numbers or letters.

Two-point discrimination

Touch two sterile needles to two places on the skin simultaneously.

Repeat the touch, moving the needles more and more

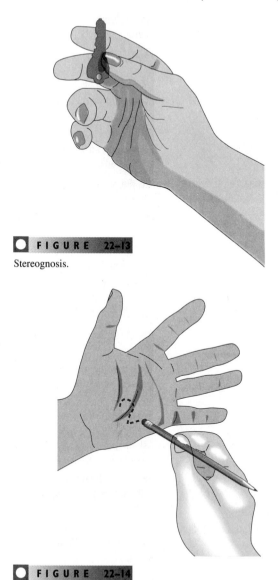

FIGURE 22-13

Stereognosis.

FIGURE 22-14

Graphesthesia.

closely together until the patient no longer feels separate points.

Record the last distance between the needles.

Extinction

Touch the same area on the right and left side of the body simultaneously.

Ask patient where and how many touches were felt.

Point location

Touch skin quickly.

Ask the patient to put the finger where the skin was just touched.

Assess reflexes

Deep tendon reflexes (DTRs)

Use a reflex hammer (Fig. 22–15) to strike the muscle's insertion tendon and thus stimulate the reflex.

Make certain the limb is relaxed but the muscle is slightly stretched.

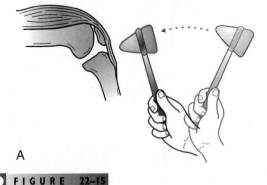

A

FIGURE 22-15

(A) Reflex hammer with motion indicated and the muscle that it is going to impact.

Illustration continued on following page

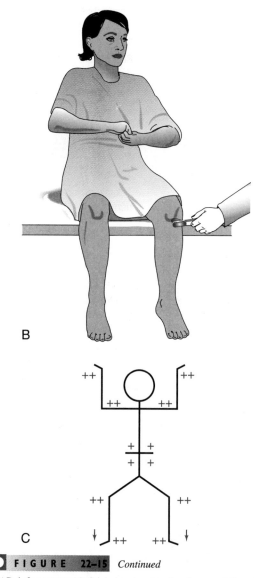

B

C

● FIGURE 22–15 *Continued*

(B) Reinforcement. *(C)* Stick drawing showing documentation of reflex activity.

Biceps reflex

Facing the patient, place the forearm to be tested over the forearm of your nondominant hand.

Place the thumb of your nondominant hand over the biceps tendon and support the patient's elbow with the rest of your hand.

Strike your thumb with the pointed end of the reflex hammer (Fig. 22–16).

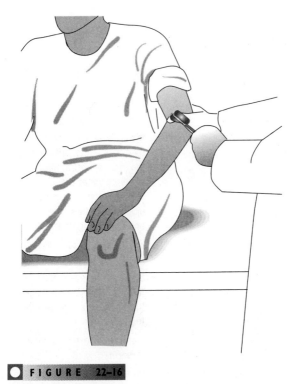

FIGURE 22–16

Testing the biceps reflex.

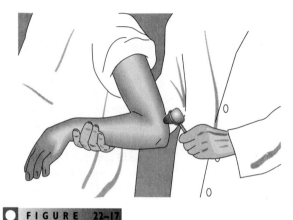

FIGURE 22-17

Testing the triceps reflex.

	Observe for flexion of the forearm.
	Repeat on other arm.
Triceps reflex	Hold the patient's arm across the chest with the elbow bent by grasping the wrist or hold the inner aspect of the patient's upper arm just above the antecubital space so the elbow is bent and the forearm and hand hang down.
	Tell the patient to let the arm go "dead."
	Strike the triceps tendon with the pointed end of the reflex hammer just above the elbow (Fig. 22–17).
	Observe for extension of the forearm.
	Repeat on patient's other arm.

Brachioradialis reflex

Have the patient rest the hands with the ulnar side down, thumb side up, in the lap.

Strike the forearm 2 to 3 cm above the radial styloid process with the pointed end of the reflex hammer (Fig. 22–18).

Observe for flexion and supination of the forearm.

Repeat on other arm.

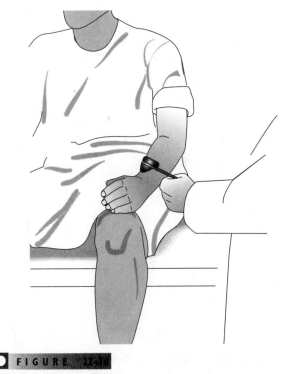

⬤ F I G U R E   22–18

Testing the brachioradialis reflex.

Patellar (knee-jerk) reflex

Ask the patient to sit and dangle the legs freely over the side of the examining table or bed.

Place your nondominant hand across the patient's leg just above the knee.

Strike the tendon just below the patella with the wide end of the reflex hammer (Fig. 22–19).

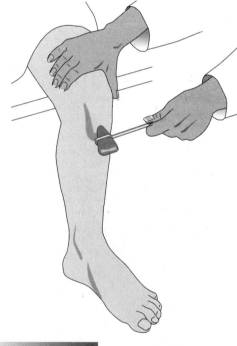

● FIGURE 22–19

Testing the patellar reflex.

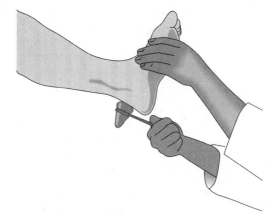

● FIGURE 22-20

Testing the achilles reflex.

Observe for extension of the lower leg and feel for contraction of the quadriceps.

If the patient is unable to sit up and dangle the legs, flex the patient's knee by placing your nondominant arm under it.

Support the weight by bracing your hand on top of the patient's other leg just above the knee.

Achilles reflex

Flex the patient's knee and externally rotate the hip, and dorsiflex the foot.

Strike the Achilles tendon with the wide end of the reflex hammer (Fig. 22-20).

Feel for plantar flexion of the foot in your hand.

Test for clonus especially if reflexes are hyperactive	Place one hand under the calf to support the lower leg.
	Dorsiflex the foot briskly with the other hand and hold it in dorsiflexion.
	Observe and feel for rapid rhythmic contractions of the foot.
Superficial reflexes (receptors in skin)	Ask the patient to lie flat on the back with the knees slightly bent.
Upper and lower abdominal	Stroke the skin with the handle of the reflex hammer, moving from the side of the abdomen into the midline. Do this on the right and left side of the upper (below the rib cage and above the umbilicus) and lower (above the symphysis pubis) abdomen (Fig. 22–21A).
	Observe for contraction of the abdominal muscle on the side stroked accompanied by deviation of the umbilicus to that same side.
	If the patient is obese, pull the skin to the opposite side and feel for it to pull back toward the side stroked.
Cremasteric reflex	Use the handle of the reflex hammer to stroke the inner aspect of the male thigh (Fig. 22–21B).
	Observe for elevation of the testicle on the side stroked.

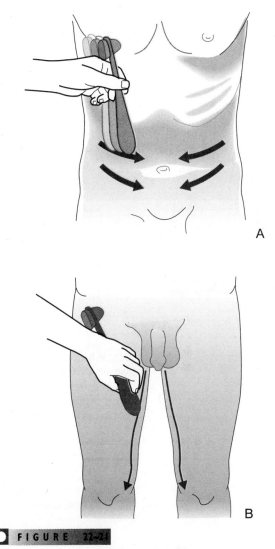

FIGURE   22-24

(A) Abdominal reflexes. *(B)* Cremasteric reflex.

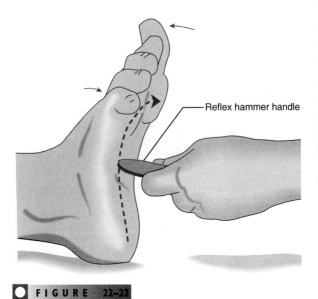

Reflex hammer handle

○ FIGURE 22-22

Plantar reflex.

Plantar reflex		Use the handle of the reflex hammer to stroke the lateral side of the sole of the foot and across the ball of the foot, forming an upside down "J" (Fig. 22–22).
		Observe for plantar flexion of toes or foot.

	Normal Findings	*Abnormal Findings*
Mental status speech and language	See Chapter 4	See Chapter 4
Expressive speech function	Follows simple directions	Unable to follow simple directions

	Responds to complex commands without demonstration	Unable to respond to complex demands without demonstration
Receptive speech function	Repeats phrases clearly, fluently	Hesitates, uses substitute words, speech unclear
	Identifies common objects correctly by name	Cannot identify common objects, or identifies by function, not name

Cranial nerve function

CN I	Common odors are correctly identified using each side of the nose	Decreased or loss of smell (anosmia) unilaterally or bilaterally
CN II	Visual field intact	Visual field loss
		Papilledema, optic atrophy
CN III, IV, VI	PERRLA	Ptosis, pupillary abnormalities (Table 22–2), deviated gaze, limited eye movement, nystagmus (other than end point)
CN V		
Motor function	Symmetric jaw movement	Asymmetric jaw movement
	Equal muscle strength on left and right sides sufficient to prevent examiner from separating jaw	Unilateral or bilateral decreased strength

Sensory function	Sensations of light touch, dullness, and sharpness perceived over forehead, cheeks, and chin	Absent, decreased, or unequal sensation
	Eyelids blink when cornea touched with cotton (also reflects motor function of CN VII)	Absent blink
CN VII		
Motor function	Symmetrical strength and movement of facial muscles	Loss of or asymmetric movement
		Muscle weakness suggested by loss of nasolabial fold, droopy side of face, or drooping of lower lid, no escape of air from one or both cheeks
Sensory function	Correctly identifies salt, sweet, sour, and bitter taste	Unable to identify salty, sweet, sour, and/or bitter taste
CN VIII	Hearing acuity within normal range	Unilateral or bilateral hearing impairment (see Chapter 8)
CN IX and X		
Motor function	Uvula and soft palate rise in midline and tonsillar pillars move medially when patient says "ah"	Absence or asymmetry of movement
		Deviated uvula

	Voice smooth	Voice hoarse or strained
	Gag reflex intact	Absence of gag reflex
CN XI	Muscle strength equal on left and right	Muscle weakness or paralysis
CN XII	Tongue is midline when protruded, lingual sounds clear, nonpurposeful movement is absent	Wasting, tremors tongue deviates to side
		Indistinct, lingual speech sounds

Motor function

Muscle mass and size	Symmetrical size (muscles on dominant side may be somewhat larger than those the nondominant side)	Unilateral or bilateral atrophy or marked hypertrophy
Muscle tone	Mild, even resistance to movement	Flacidity, decreased resistance, spasticity, rigidity
Movement	Equal on both sides, normal range of motion	Limited movement bilaterally or unilaterally
Muscle strength	Approximately equal on both sides	Marked asymmetric strength

Balance and coordination

Gait	Smooth, rhythmic, effortless swing of arms coordinated with step of opposite legs, able	Stiffness, staggering, reeling, lack of arm swing, unequal rhythm of steps, abnormally

	to walk a straight line	wide base of support, scraping of toe or slapping of foot on floor
		Inability to walk a straight line
Romberg's test	Position maintained with no more than slight swaying	Swaying, falling, weakening of base of support
Rapid alternating movements	Rapid, smooth, accurate movement	Slow, clumsy, jerky, uncoordinated movement
Arm drift	No drift	Downward drift or pronation
Finger-to-finger test	Smooth, accurate movement	Misses the nose or finger
Finger-to-nose test	Smooth, accurate movement	Misses nose, jerky movements
Heel-to-shin test	Smoothly moves heel in a straight line down the shin	Heel falls off shin
Sensory function		
Light touch	Touch sensation intact	Increased, decreased or absent touch sensation
Superficial pain sensation	Sensations are correctly identified as sharp or dull	Sensations are not perceived or are incorrectly identified as sharp or dull
Temperature sensitivity	Hot and cold temperatures are correctly identified	Inability to distinguish hot from cold
Position sense	Direction of digit	Digit movement

	movement is correctly identified	not detected
Vibration sense	Vibration perceived equally	Vibration not perceived
Stereognosis	Object is correctly named	Object is not correctly named
Graphesthesia	Number is correctly identified	Number is not correctly identified
Two-point discrimination	2 to 8mm in fingertips 40 to 75 mm on upper arms, thighs, and back	Increase in minimal distance at which two points are perceived
Extinction	Sensations felt on both sides of the body	Absent or unilateral sensation
Point location	Area of skin touched can be identified	Area of skin touched unable to be identified
Deep tendon reflexes		
Biceps reflex	Flexion of the forearm	Hypo- or hyperreflexia
Triceps reflex	Extension of the forearm	Hypo- or hyperreflexia
Brachioradialis reflex	Flexion and supination of the forearm	Hypo- or hyperreflexia
Quadriceps reflex	Extension of the lower leg	Hypo- or hyperreflexia
Achilles reflex	Plantar flexion of the foot	Hypo- or hyperreflexia
Clonus	No movement	Rapid rhythmic contractions of the foot

Superficial reflexes	Ipsilateral contraction of the abdominal muscle accompanied by	Absence of muscular contraction
Upper and lower abdominal reflex	deviation of the umbilicus toward the stimulated side	
Cremasteric reflex	Ipsilateral elevation of the testicle	Absence of testicular elevation
Plantar reflex	Plantar flexion of the toes or foot	Dorsiflexion of the great toe and fanning of all toes (positive Babinski sign)

Clinical Note

To determine changes in neurologic baseline quickly assess as follows:

Level of consciousness	Assess orientation to person, place, time, and reality.
	Assess appropriateness of speech; note clarity and fluency.
Cranial nerves	Assess pupillary response to light bilaterally (oculomotor nerve).
	Assess extraocular movements: oculomotor, trochlear, and abducens nerves.
	Assess facial symmetry (facial nerve).
	Assess gag reflex (glossopharyngeal nerve).
	Assess tongue in midline when extended (hypoglossal nerve).
Motor function	Assess arm drifting.
	Assess handgrip.
	Assess straight-leg raise.
	Assess knee bends.

Assess ankle plantar flexion and dorsiflexion.

Sensory function   Assess sensation to light touch and pin-
prick in extremities and on trunk, com-
paring right with left sides.

Geriatric Considerations

Normal Findings

Reflexes   Reaction time and response to
stimuli slowed. Gag, ankle,
abdominal and plantar reflexes
may be diminished or absent.

Also see geriatric considerations in Chapters 3, 6, and 20.

Clinical Note

Changes of the nervous system attributable to aging are
generally symmetrical. If asymmetric, investigate for cause
other than aging.

Pediatric Considerations

History

Pregnancy and birth history?
Quality of cry?
Developmental history: meeting age-appropriate
milestones?
Abnormal sucking or eye movements?
"Absence" spells?
Accident, injuries, ingestions?
Family history of metabolic, genetic, or any progressive
neurologic condition? Seizure disorders?

Physical Examination

Observe for newborn reflexes, then age-appropriate sup-
pression
Note infant's level of alertness and arousability
Note infant's position/posturing
Test vision and hearing in the age-appropriate manner

Equipment

Bell

Findings

Normal Findings	Common Variations	Abnormal Findings
Newborn		
Crying but consolable	Intermittent fussiness	Extreme irritability, not consolable
		High-pitched "cat's cry"
Newborn reflexes present:	Disappears at approximately:	Newborn reflexes asymmetric, absent, or persisting beyond expected time of disappearance
Crawling	1–2 mos	
Dance	1–2 mos	
Tonic neck	4–6 mos	
Moro	4–6 mos	
Grasp (palmer and plantar)	3–4 mos	
+ Babinski	1–2 yrs	
Rooting and sucking	3–4 mos	
Neck righting	10 mos	
Symmetric muscle tone, bulk, and movement; rapid recoil after extension	Fine tremors of short duration	Asymmetry
	Ankle clonus	Flaccidity
		Tremors that cannot be quieted by the examiner
		Stiffness
		Extension
		Spastic adduction
		Athetosis

Fontanelles soft and flat	Various sizes	Bulging or markedly depressed
Hearing: May respond by opening eyes wide, blinking, ceasing or initiating movement, or turning to sound		No response

Infant

Reflexes

Neck righting (4–6 mos)

Parachute (8–9 mos)

Separation anxiety when removed from primary caretaker (9 mos)

Child

Cerebral dominance (3–4 yrs)

| Clear speech (90% understandable other than by primary caretaker) | | Unclear speech |

Appendix 1
Height and Weight Table

1983 Metropolitan Life Table*

Men

Height Feet	Height Inches	Small frame	Medium frame	Large frame
5	2	128-134	131-141	138-150
5	3	130-136	133-143	140-153
5	4	132-138	135-145	142-156
5	5	134-140	137-148	144-160
5	6	136-142	139-151	146-164
5	7	138-145	142-154	149-168
5	8	140-148	145-157	152-172
5	9	142-151	148-160	155-176
5	10	144-154	151-163	158-180
5	11	146-157	154-166	161-184
6	0	149-160	157-170	164-188
6	1	152-164	160-174	168-192

Women

Height Feet	Height Inches	Small frame	Medium frame	Large frame
4	10	102-111	109-121	118-131
4	11	103-113	111-123	120-134
5	0	104-115	113-126	122-137
5	1	106-118	115-129	125-140
5	2	108-121	118-132	128-143
5	3	111-124	121-135	131-147
5	4	114-127	124-138	134-151
5	5	117-130	127-141	137-155
5	6	120-133	130-144	140-159
5	7	123-136	133-147	143-163
5	8	126-139	133-150	146-167
5	9	129-142	139-153	149-170

1983 Metropolitan Life Table* *(Continued)*

Men

Height		Small frame	Medium frame	Large frame
Feet	Inches			
6	2	155-168	164-178	172-197
6	3	158-172	167-182	176-202
6	4	162-176	171-187	181-207

Women

Height		Small frame	Medium frame	Large frame
Feet	Inches			
5	10	132-145	142-156	152-173
5	11	135-148	145-159	155-176
6	0	138-151	148-162	158-179

From Society of Actuaries, Build Study, 1979, Chicago, 1980. Society of Actuaries and Association of Life Insurance Medical Directors of America, Metropolitan Life Insurance Co., New York, 1983. Courtesy Statistical Bulletin, Metropolitan Life Insurance, New York.

Weight in pounds at ages 29 to 59 years according to build. In shoes and 3 lb of indoor clothing for women and 5 lb for men.

GIRLS: BIRTH TO 36 MONTHS
PHYSICAL GROWTH
NCHS PERCENTILES*

NAME _____   RECORD # _____

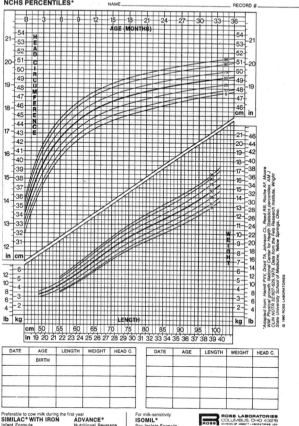

DATE	AGE	LENGTH	WEIGHT	HEAD C.
	BIRTH			

DATE	AGE	LENGTH	WEIGHT	HEAD C.

Preferable to cow milk during the first year
SIMILAC® WITH IRON   ADVANCE®
Infant Formula   Nutritional Beverage

For milk-sensitivity
ISOMIL®
Soy Isolate Formula

ROSS LABORATORIES
COLUMBUS, OHIO 43216
DIVISION OF ABBOTT LABORATORIES USA

G106 January 1980

*Adapted from: Hamill PVV, Drizd TA, Johnson CL, Reed RB, Roche AF, Moore WM: Physical growth: National Center for Health Statistics percentiles. AM J CLIN NUTR 32:607-629, 1979. Data from the Fels Research Institute, Wright State University School of Medicine, Yellow Springs, Ohio.
© 1980 ROSS LABORATORIES

GIRLS PREPUBESCENT
**PHYSICAL GROWTH
NCHS PERCENTILES***

Name_____ Record #_____

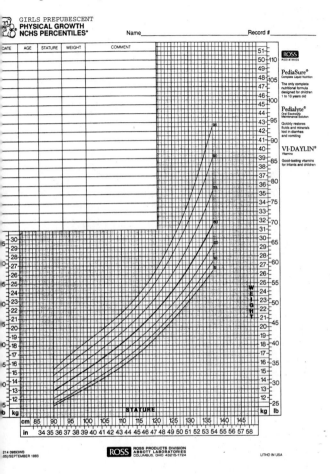

DATE	AGE	STATURE	WEIGHT	COMMENT

214 09893WB
.05)/SEPTEMBER 1993

ROSS ROSS PRODUCTS DIVISION
ABBOTT LABORATORIES
COLUMBUS, OHIO 43215-1724

LITHO IN USA

BOYS: BIRTH TO 36 MONTHS
PHYSICAL GROWTH
NCHS PERCENTILES*

NAME _____   RECORD # _____

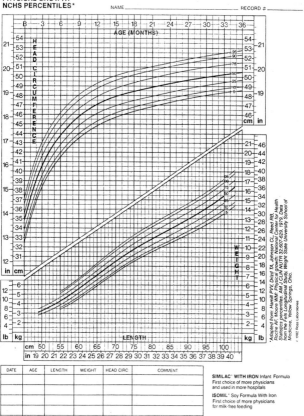

DATE	AGE	LENGTH	WEIGHT	HEAD CIRC	COMMENT

SIMILAC® WITH IRON Infant Formula
First choice of more physicians
and used in more hospitals

ISOMIL® Soy Formula With Iron
First choice of more physicians
for milk-free feeding

ROSS LABORATORIES
COLUMBUS, OHIO 43216
Division of Abbott Laboratories, USA

51256 0949/WB
(0.05) OCTOBER 1992   LITHO IN USA

BOYS: PREPUBESCENT
PHYSICAL GROWTH
NCHS PERCENTILES*

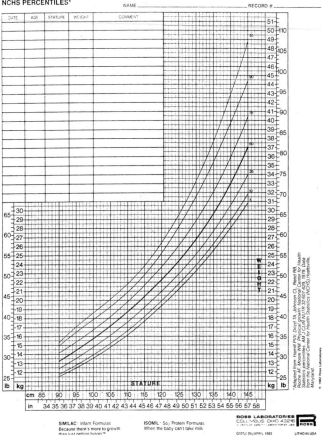

Appendix 2
Temperature Table

**Temperature Conversion Table
(Centigrade to Fahrenheit)**

Celsius (C°)	Fahrenheit (F°)	Celsius (C°)	Fahrenheit (F°)
34.0	93.2	38.6	101.4
34.2	93.6	38.8	101.8
34.4	93.9	39.0	102.2
34.6	94.3	39.2	102.5
34.8	94.6	39.4	102.9
35.0	95.0	39.6	103.2
35.2	95.4	39.8	103.6
35.4	95.7	40.0	104.0
35.6	96.1	40.2	104.3
35.8	96.4	40.4	104.7
36.0	96.8	40.6	105.1
36.2	97.1	40.8	105.4
36.4	97.5	41.0	105.8
36.6	97.8	41.2	106.1
36.8	98.2	41.4	106.5
37.0	98.6	41.6	106.8
37.2	98.9	41.8	107.2
37.4	99.3	42.0	107.6
37.6	99.6	42.2	108.0
37.8	100.0	42.4	108.3
38.0	100.4	42.6	108.7

Continued

Temperature Conversion Table (Centigrade to Fahrenheit)

Celsius (C°)	Fahrenheit (F°)	Celsius (C°)	Fahrenheit (F°)
38.2	100.7	42.8	109.0
38.4	101.0	43.0	109.4

Conversion of Celsius (Centigrade) to Fahrenheit:
($9/5 \times$ temperature + 32)

Conversion of Fahrenheit to Celsius (Centigrade):
(Temperature − 32) × 5/9

From Monahan, F.D. & Neighbors, M. Pocket Companion for Nursing Code of Adults. Philadelphia; WB Saunders, 1994. Appendix 2 pp. 474–475.

Appendix 3

Daily Requirements of Basic Food Groups

Daily Requirements of Basic Food Groups

How many servings do you need each day?

	Women & some older adults	Children, teen girls, active women, most men	Teen boys & active men
Calorie level*	about 1,600	about 2,200	about 2,800
Bread group	6	9	11
Vegetable group	3	4	5
Fruit group	2	3	4

Continued

Daily Requirements of Basic Food Groups
(Continued)

How many servings do you need each day?

Milk group	**2–3	**2–3	**2–3
Meat group	2, for a total of 5 ounces	2, for a total of 6 ounces	3, for a total of 7 ounces

*These are the calorie levels if you choose lowfat, lean foods from the 5 major food groups and use foods from the fats, oils, and sweets group sparingly.

**Women who are pregnant or breastfeeding, teenagers, and young adults to age 24 need 3 servings.

Appendix 4

Normal Laboratory Values

Reference Values in Hematology

	Conventional Units	SI Units
Acid hemolysis test (Ham)	No hemolysis	No hemolysis
Alkaline phosphatase, leukocyte	Total score 14–100	Total score 14–100
Cell counts		
Erythrocytes		
Males	4.6–6.2 million/mm^3	4.6–6.2 × 10^{12}/L
Females	4.2–5.4 million/mm^3	4.2–5.4 × 10^{12}/L
Children (varies with age)	4.5–5.1 million/mm^3	4.5–5.1 × 10^{12}/L
Leukocytes		
Total	4500–11,000 mm^3	4.5–11.0 × 10^9/L
Differential	*Percentage*	*Absolute*	*Absolute*
Myelocytes	0	0/mm^3	0/L
Band neutrophils	3–5	150–400/mm^3	150–400 × 10^6/L
Segmented neutrophils	54–62	3000–5800/mm^3	3000–5800 × 10^6/L
Lymphocytes	25–33	1500–3000/mm^3	1500–3000 × 10^6/L
Monocytes	3–7	300–500/mm^3	300–500 × 10^6/L
Eosinophils	1–3	50–250/mm^3	50–250 × 10^6/L
Basophils	0–0.75	15–50/mm^3	15–50 × 10^6/L
Platelets		150,000–350,000/mm^3	150–350 × 10^9/L

Continued

Reference Values in Hematology (Continued)

	Conventional Units	SI Units
Reticulocytes	25,000–75,000/mm³	25–75 × 10⁹/L
	0.5–1.5% of erythrocytes	
Coagulation tests		
Bleeding time (template)	2.75–8.0 min	2.75–8.0 min
Coagulation time (glass tubes)	5–15 min	5–15 min
Factor VIII and other coagulation factors	50–150% of normal	0.5–1.5 of normal
Fibrin split products (Thrombo-Welco test)	<10 µg/mL	<10 mg/L
Fibrinogen	200–400 mg/dL	2.0–4.0 g/L
Partial thromboplastin time (PTT)	20–35 sec	20–35 s
Prothrombin time (PT)	12.0–14.0 sec	12.0–14.0 s
Coombs' test		
Direct	Negative	Negative
Indirect	Negative	Negative
Corpuscular values of erythrocytes		
Mean corpuscular hemoglobin (MCH)	26–34 pg	0.40–0.53 fmol
Mean corpuscular volume (MCV)	80–96 µm³	80–96 fL
Mean corpuscular hemoglobin concentration (MCHC)	32–36%	0.32–0.36
Haptoglobin	26–185 mg/dL	260–1850 mg/L

Hematocrit		
Males	40–54 mL/dL	0.40–0.54 volume fraction
Females	37–47 mL/dL	0.37–0.47 volume fraction
Newborns	49–54 mL/dL	0.49–0.54 volume fraction
Children (varies with age)	35–49 mL/dL	0.35–0.49 volume fraction
Hemoglobin		
Males	14.0–18.0 gm/dL	2.17–2.79 mmol/L
Females	12.0–16.0 gm/dL	1.86–2.48 mmol/L
Newborns	16.5–19.5 gm/dL	2.56–3.02 mmol/L
Children (varies with age)	11.2–16.5 gm/dL	1.74–2.56 mmol/L
Hemoglobin, fetal	<1.0% of total	<0.01 of total
Hemoglobin A_{1C}	3–5% of total	0.03–0.05 of total
Hemoglobin A_2	1.5–3.0% of total	0.015–0.03 of total
Hemoglobin, plasma	0–5.0 mg/dL	0–0.8 µmol/L
Methemoglobin	30–130 mg/dL	4.7–20 µmol/L
Sedimentation rate (ESR)		
Wintrobe: Males	0–5 mm/hr	0–5 mm/h
Females	0–15 mm/hr	0–15 mm/h
Westergren: Males	0–15 mm/hr	0–15 mm/h
Females	0–20 mm/hr	0–20 mm/h

Reference Values for Blood, Plasma, and Serum*

	Conventional Units	SI Units
Acetoacetate plus acetone, serum		
Qualitative	Negative	Negative
Quantitative	0.3–2.0 mg/dL	3–20 mg/L
Acid phosphatase (thymolphthalein monophosphate substrate), serum	0.11–0.60 U/L	0.11–0.60 U/L
Adrenocorticotropin (ACTH), plasma		
6 A.M.	10–80 pg/mL	10–80 ng/L
6 P.M.	<50 pg/mL	<50 ng/L
Alanine aminotransferase (ALT, SGPT), serum	5–30 U/L	5–30 U/L
Albumin, serum	3.5–5.5 gm/dL	35–55 g/L
Aldolase, serum	1.5–12.0 U/L	1.5–12.0 U/L
Aldosterone, plasma		
Supine	3–10 ng/dL	0.08–0.30 nmol/L
Standing		
Males	6–22 ng/dL	0.17–0.61 nmol/L
Females	5–30 ng/dL	0.14–0.83 nmol/L
Alkaline phosphatase (ALP), serum	20–90 U/L (30°C)	20–90 U/L (30°C)
Ammonia nitrogen, plasma	15–49 μg/dL	11–35 μmol/L
Amylase, serum	25–125 U/L	25–125 U/L
Anion gap	8–16 mEq/L	8–16 mmol/L
Ascorbic acid, blood	0.4–1.5 mg/dL	23–85 μmol/L
Aspartate aminotransferase (AST, SGOT), serum	10–30 U/L	10–30 U/L

Base excess, blood	0 ± 2 mEq/L	0 ± 2 mmol/L
Bicarbonate		
Venous plasma	23–29 mEq/L	23–29 mmol/L
Arterial blood	18–23 mEq/L	18–23 mmol/L
Bile acids, serum	0.3–3.0 mg/dL	3–30 mg/L
Bilirubin, serum		
Conjugated	0.1–0.4 mg/dL	1.7–6.8 µmol/L
Unconjugated	0.2–0.7 mg/dL	3.4–12 µmol/L
Total	0.3–1.1 mg/dL	5.1–19 µmol/L
Calcium, serum	9.0–11.0 mg/dL	2.25–2.75 mmol/L
Calcium, ionized, serum	4.25–5.25 mg/dL	1.05–1.30 mmol/L
Carbon dioxide, total, serum or plasma	24–30 mEq/L	24–30 mmol/L
Carbon dioxide tension (P_{CO_2}), blood	35–45 mmHg	35–45 mmHg
β-Carotene, serum	40–200 µg/dL	0.74–3.72 µmol/L
Ceruloplasmin, serum	23–44 mg/dL	230–44 mg/L
Chloride, serum or plasma	96–106 mEq/L	96–106 mmol/L
Cholesterol, serum or EDTA plasma		
Desirable range	<200 mg/dL	<5.18 mmol/L
LDL cholesterol	60–180 mg/dL	600–1800 mg/L
HDL cholesterol	30–80 mg/dL	300–800 mg/L
Copper		
Males	70–140 µg/dL	11–22 µmol/L
Females	85–155 µg/dL	13–24 µmol/L

Continued

For some procedures, the reference values may vary depending on the method used.

Reference Values for Blood, Plasma, and Serum (Continued)

	Conventional Units	SI Units
Cortisol, plasma		
8 A.M.	6–23 µg/dL	170–635 nmol/L
4 P.M.	3–15 µg/dL	82–413 nmol/L
10 P.M.	<50% of 8 A.M. value	<0.5 of 8 A.M. value
Creatine, serum	0.2–0.8 mg/dL	15–61 µmol/L
Creatine kinase (CK, CPK), serum		
Males	55–170 U/L	55–170 U/L
Females	30–135 U/L	30–135 U/L
Creatine kinase MB isozyme, serum	0.0–4.7 ng/mL	0.0–4.7 µg/L
Creatinine, serum	0.6–1.2 mg/dL	53–106 µmol/L
Ferritin, serum	20–200 ng/mL	20–200 µg/L
Fibrinogen, plasma	200–400 mg/dL	2.0–4.0 g/L
Folate, serum	1.8–9.0 ng/mL	4.1–20.4 nmol/L
Erythrocytes	150–450 ng/mL	340–1020 nmol/L
Follicle-stimulating hormone (FSH), plasma		
Males	4–25 mU/mL	4–25 U/L
Females	4–30 mU/mL	4–30 U/L
Postmenopausal	40–250 mU/mL	40–250 U/L

γ-Glutamyltransferase, serum		
Males	5–38 U/L	5–38 U/L
Females	5–29 U/L	5–29 U/L
Gastrin, serum	0–200 pg/mL	0–200 ng/L
Glucose (fasting), plasma or serum	70–115 mg/dL	3.89–6.38 mmol/L
Growth hormone (hGH), plasma	0–10 ng/mL	0–10 µg/L
Haptoglobin, serum	26–185 mg/dL	260–1850 mg/L
Immunoglobulins, serum		
IgG	550–1900 mg/dL	5.5–19.0 g/L
IgA	60–333 mg/dL	0.60–3.3 g/L
IgM	45–145 mg/dL	0.45–1.5 g/L
IgD	0.5–3.0 mg/dL	5–30 mg/L
IgE	<500 ng/mL	<500 µg/L
Insulin (fasting), plasma	5–25 µU/mL	36–179 pmol/L
Iron, serum	75–175 µg/dL	13–31 µmol/L
Iron binding capacity, serum		
Total	250–410 µg/dL	45–73 µmol/L
Saturation	20–55%	0.20–0.55
Lactate		
Venous blood	4.5–19.8 mg/dL	0.50–2.2 mmol/L
Arterial blood	4.5–14.4 mg/dL	0.50–1.6 mmol/L
Lactate dehydrogenase (LD, LDH), serum	100–190 U/L	100–190 U/L

Continued

Reference Values for Blood, Plasma, and Serum (Continued)

	Conventional Units	SI Units
Lipase, serum	10–140 U/L	10–140 U/L
Lipids, total, serum	450–850 mg/dL	4.5–8.5 g/L
Luteinizing (LH), serum		
Males	6–18 IU/L	6–18 U/L
Females		
Premenopausal	5–22 IU/L	5–22 U/L
Mid-cycle	3 times baseline	3 times baseline
Postmenopausal	>30 IU/L	>30 U/L
Magnesium, serum	1.8–3.0 mg/dL	0.75–1.25 mmol/L
Osmolality	286–295 mOsm/kg water	285–295 mmol/kg water
Oxygen, blood		
Capacity (varies with hemoglobin)	16–24 vol %	
Content, arterial	15–23 vol %	
Saturation, arterial	94–100 %	0.94–1.00
Oxygen tension (Po_2), blood	75–100 mmHg	75–100 mmHg
P_{50}	26–27 mmHg	26–27 mmHg
pH, arterial blood	7.35–7.45	7.35–7.45
Phenylalanine, serum	<3 mg/dL	<0.18 mmol/L
Phosphate, inorganic, serum	3.0–4.5 mg/dL	1.0–1.5 mmol/L

Potassium, serum or plasma	3.5–5.0 mEq/L	3.5–5.0 mmol/L
Prolactin		
Males	1–20 ng/mL	1–20 μg/L
Females	1–25 ng/mL	1–25 μg/L
Protein, serum		
Total	6.0–8.0 gm/dL	60–80 g/L
Albumin	3.5–5.5 gm/dL	35–55 g/L
Alpha$_1$ globulin	0.2–0.4 gm/dL	2–4 g/L
Alpha$_2$ globulin	0.5–0.9 gm/dL	5–9 g/L
Beta globulin	0.6–1.1 gm/dL	6–11 g/L
Gamma globulin	0.7–1.7 gm/dL	7–17 g/L
Pyruvate, blood	0.3–0.9 mg/dL	0.03–0.10 mmol/L
Sodium, serum or plasma	136–145 mEq/L	136–145 mmol/L
Testosterone, plasma		
Males	275–875 ng/dL	9.5–30 nmol/L
Females	23–75 ng/dL	0.8–2.6 nmol/L
Pregnant	38–190 ng/dL	1.3–6.6 nmol/L
Thyroid-stimulating hormone (TSH), serum	0–7 μU/mL	0–7 mU/L
Thyroxine, free (FT), serum	1.0–2.1 ng/dL	13–27 pmol/L
Thyroxine (T$_4$), serum	4.4–9.9 μg/dL	57–128 nmol/L
Triglycerides, serum	40–150 mg/dL	0.4–1.5 g/L
Triiodothyronine (T$_3$), serum	150–250 ng/dL	2.3–3.9 nmol/L
Triiodothyronine uptake, resin (T$_3$RU)	25–38% uptake	0.25–0.38 uptake

Continued

Reference Values for Blood, Plasma, and Serum *(Continued)*

	Conventional Units	SI Units
Urate, serum		
Males	2.5–8.0 mg/dL	0.15–0.48 mmol/L
Females	1.5–7.0 mg/dL	0.09–0.42 mmol/L
Urea, serum or plasma	24–49 mg/dL	4.0–8.2 mmol/L
Urea nitrogen, serum or plasma	11–23 mg/dL	3.9–8.2 mmol/L
Viscosity, serum	1.4–1.8 times water	1.4–1.8 times water
Vitamin A, serum	20–80 µg/dL	0.70–2.80 µmol/L
Vitamin B_{12}, serum	180–900 pg/mL	133–664 pmol/L

Reference Values for Urine*

	Conventional Units	SI Units
Acetone and acetoacetate, qualitative	Negative	Negative
Albumin		
Qualitative	Negative	Negative
Quantitative	10–100 mg/24 hr	0.15–1.5 μmol/24 h
Aldosterone	3–20 μg/24 hr	8.3–55 nmol/24 h
δ-Aminolevulinic acid	1.3–7.0 mg/24 hr	10–53 μmol/24 h
Amylase	3–20 U/hr	3–20 U/h
Amylase/creatinine clearance ratio	1–4%	0.01–0.04
Bilirubin, qualitative	Negative	Negative
Calcium (usual diet)	<250 mg/24 hr	<6.3 mmol/24 h
Catecholamines		
Epinephrine	<10 μg/24 hr	<55 nmol/24 h
Norepinephrine	<100 μg/24 hr	<590 nmol/24 h
Total free catecholamines	4–126 μg/24 hr	24–745 nmol/24 h
Total metanephrines	0.1–1.6 mg/24 hr	0.5–8.1 μmol/24 h
Chloride (varies with intake)	110–250 mEq/24 hr	110–250 mmol/24 h
Copper	0–50 μg/24 hr	0–0.80 μmol/24 h

For some procedures, the reference values may vary depending on the method used.

Continued

Reference Values for Urine* (Continued)

Cortisol, free	10–100 µg/24 hr	27.6–276 nmol/24 h
Creatinine	15–25 mg/kg body weight in/24 hr	0.13–0.22 mmol/kg body weight/24 h
Creatinine clearance (corrected to 1.73 m² body surface area)		
Males	110–150 mL/min	110–150 ml/min
Females	105–132 mL/min	105–132 ml/min
Dehydroepiandrosterone		
Males	0.2–2.0 mg/24 hr	0.7–6.9 µmol/24 h
Females	0.2–1.8 mg/24 hr	0.7–6.2 µmol/24 h
Estrogens, total		
Males	4–25 µg/24 hr	14–90 nmol/24 h
Females	5–100 µg/24 hr	18–360 nmol/24 h
Glucose (as reducing substance)	<250 mg/24 hr	<250 mg/24 h
Hemoglobin and myoglobin, qualitative	Negative	Negative
17-Hydroxycorticosteroids		
Males	3–9 mg/24 hr	8.3–25 µmol/24 h
Females	2–8 mg/24 hr	5.5–22 µmol/24 h
5-Hydroxyindoleacetic acid		
Qualitative	Negative	Negative
Quantitative	<9 mg/24 hr	<47 µmol/24 h

17-Ketosteroids		
Males	6–18 mg/24 hr	21–62 μmol/24 h
Females	4–13 mg/24 hr	14–45 μmol/24 h
Magnesium	6.0–8.5 mEq/24 hr	3.0–4.2 mmol/24 h
Metanephrines (see Catecholamines)		
Osmolality	38–1400 mOsm/kg water	38–1400 mmol/kg water
pH	4.6–8.0	4.6–8.0
Phenylpyruvic acid, qualitative	Negative	Negative
Phosphate	0.9–1.3 grams/24 hr	29–42 mmol/24 h
Porphobilinogen		
Qualitative	Negative	Negative
Quantitative	<2.0 mg/24 hr	<9 μmol/24 h
Porphyrins		
Coproporphyrin	50–250 μg/24 hr	77–380 nmol/24 h
Uroporphyrin	10–30 μg/24 hr	12–36 nmol/24 h
Potassium	25–100 mEq/24 hr	25–100 mmol/24 h
Pregnanediol		
Males	0.4–1.4 mg/24 hr	1.2–4.4 μmol/24 h
Females		
Proliferative phase	0.5–1.5 mg/24 hr	1.6–4.7 μmol/24 h
Luteal phase	2.0–7.0 mg/24 hr	6.2–22 μmol/24 h
Postmenopausal	0.2–1.0 mg/24 hr	0.6–3.1 μmol/24 h
Pregnanetriol	<2.5 mg/24 hr	<7.4 μmol/24 h

Continued

Reference Values for Urine* *(Continued)*

Protein		
Qualitative	Negative	Negative
Quantitative	10–150 mg/24 hr	10–150 mg/24 h
Sodium	130–260 mEq/24 hr	130–260 mmol/24 h
Specific gravity	1.003–1.030	1.003–1.030
Urate	200–500 mg/24 hr	1.2–3.0 mmol/24 h
Urobilinogen	<4.0 mg/24 hr	<6.8 µmol/24 h
Vanillylmandelic acid (VMA, 4-hydroxy-3-methoxymandelic acid)	1–8 mg/24 hr	5–40 µmol/24 h

Reference Values for Therapeutic Drug Monitoring

	Therapeutic Range	Toxic Levels	Proprietary Names
ANTIBIOTICS			
Amikacin, serum	25–30 μg/mL	Peak: >35 μg/mL Trough: >5–7 μg/mL	Amikin
Chloramphenicol, serum	10–20 μg/mL	>25 μg/mL	Chloromycetin
Gentamicin, serum	5–10 μg/mL	Peak: >12 μg/mL Trough: >12 μg/mL	Garamycin
Tobramycin, serum	5–10 μg/mL	Peak: >12 μg/mL Trough: >2 μg/mL	Nebcin
ANTICONVULSANTS			
Carbamazepine, serum	5-12 μg/mL	>12 μg/mL	Tegretol
Ethosuximide, serum	40–100 μg/mL	>100 μg/mL	Zarontin
Phenobarbital, serum	10–30 μg/mL	Vary widely because of developed tolerance	
Phenytoin, serum	10–20 μg/mL	>20 μg/mL	Dilantin
Primidone, serum	5-12 μg/mL	>15 μg/mL	Mysoline
Valproic acid, serum	50–100 μg/mL	>100 μg/mL	Depakene

Continued

Reference Values for Therapeutic Drug Monitoring

	Therapeutic Range	Toxic Levels	Proprietary Names
ANALGESICS			
Acetaminophen, serum	10–20 µg/mL	>250 µg/mL	Tylenol
Salicylate, serum	100–250 µg/mL	>300 µg/mL	Disalcid
BRONCHODILATOR			
Theophylline (aminophylline), serum	10–20 µg/mL	>20 µg/mL	
CARDIOVASCULAR DRUGS			
Digitoxin, serum (specimen must be obtained 12–24 hr after last dose)	15–25 ng/mL	>25 ng/mL	Crystodigin
Digoxin, serum (specimen must be obtained 12–24 hr after last dose)	0.8–2.0 ng/mL	>2.4 ng/mL	Lanoxin
Disopyramide, serum	2–5 µg/mL	>5 µg/mL	Norpace
Lidocaine, serum	1.5–5.0 µg/mL	>6–8 µg/mL	Xylocaine
Procainamide, serum (measured as procainamide + N-acetylprocainamide)	4–10 µg/mL	>16 µg/mL	Pronestyl
Propranolol, serum	50–100 ng/mL	Variable	Inderal
Quinidine, serum	2–5 µg/mL	>10 µg/mL	Cardioquin Quinaglute Quinidex Quinora

PSYCHOPHARMACOLOGIC DRUGS

Amitriptyline, serum (measured as amitriptyline + nortriptyline)	120–150 ng/mL	>500 ng/mL	Amitril Elavil Endep Limbitrol Triavil
Desipramine, serum (measured as desipramine + imipramine)	150–300 ng/mL	>500 ng/mL	Norpramin Pertofrane
Imipramine, serum (measured as imipramine + desipramine)	150–300 ng/mL	>500 ng/mL	Antipress Imavate Janimine Presamine Tofranil
Lithium, serum (obtain specimen 12 hr after last dose)	0.8–1.2 mEq/L	>2.0 mEq/L	Lithobid
Nortriptyline, serum	50–150 ng/mL	>500 ng/mL	Aventyl Pamelor

Reference Values in Toxicology

	Conventional Units	SI Units
Arsenic		
Blood	3.5–7.2 µg/dL	0.47–0.96 µmol/L
Urine	<100 µg/24 hr	<1.3 µmol/24 h
Bromides, serum	0	0
Carboxyhemoglobin, blood	Toxic: >17 mEq/L	Toxic: >17 mmol/L
Symptoms occur	<5% saturation	<0.05 saturation
	>20% saturation	>0.20 saturation
Ethanol, blood	<0.05 mg/dL (<0.005%)	<1.0 mmol/L
Marked intoxication	300–400 mg/dL (0.3–0.4%)	65–87 mmol/L
Alcoholic stupor	400–500 mg/dL (0.4–0.5%)	87–109 mmol/L
Coma	>500 mg/dL (0.5%)	>109 mmol/L
Lead		
Blood	0–40 µg/dL	0–2 µmol/L
Urine	<100 µg/24 hr	<0.48 µmol/24 h
Mercury, urine	<100 µg/24 hr	<50 nmol/L

Reference Values for Cerebrospinal Fluid

	Conventional Units	SI Units
Cells	<5/mm³; all mononuclear	<5 × 10⁶/L, all mononuclear
Electrophoresis	Predominantly albumin	Predominantly albumin
Glucose	50–75 mg/dL	2.8–4.2 mmol/L
	(20 mg/dL less than serum)	(1.1 mmol less than serum)
IgG		
Children under 14	<8% of total protein	<0.08 of total protein
Adults	<14% of total protein	<0.14 of total protein
IgG index $\left(\dfrac{\text{CSF/serum IgG ratio}}{\text{CSF/serum albumin ratio}} \right)$	0.3–0.6	0.3–0.6
Oligoclonal banding on electrophoresis	Absent	Absent
Pressure	70–180 mm water	70–180 mm water
Protein, total	15–45 mg/dL	150–450 mg/L

Reference Values for Semen

	Conventional Units	SI Units
Volume	2–5 mL	2–5 mL
Liquefaction	Complete in 15 min	Complete in 15 min
Leukocytes	Occasional or absent	Occasional or absent
Count	60–150 million/mL	$60–150 \times 10^6$/mL
Motility	>80% motile	>0.80 motile
Morphology	80–90% normal forms	0.80–0.90 normal forms
Fructose	>150 mg/dL	>8.33 mmol/L

Reference Values for Feces

	Conventional Units	SI Units
Bulk	100–200 gm/24 hr	100–200 g/24 h
Dry matter	23–32 gm/24 hr	23–32 g/24 h
Fat, total	<6.0 gm/24 hr	<6.0 g/24 h
Nitrogen, total	<2.0 gm/24 hr	<2.0 g/24 h
Water	Approximately 65%	Approximately 0.65

Tables from Rakel RE (ed). Conn's current therapy. Philadelphia; WB Saunders, 1992. Reference Values for Laboratory Tests.

Appendix 5

Glasgow Coma Scale

Variable	Response	Scale No.
Eyes	Open spontaneously	4
	Open to verbal commands	3
	Open to pain	2
	No response	1
Best motor response	Obeys verbal command	6
	To painful stimulus	
	Localizes pain	5
	Flexion withdrawal	4
	Flexion abnormal	3
	Extension	2
	No response	1
Best verbal response	Oriented and converses	5
	Disoriented and converses	4
	Inappropriate words	3
	Incomprehensible sounds	2
	No response	1
Total		3–15

Appendix 6
Dermatomes

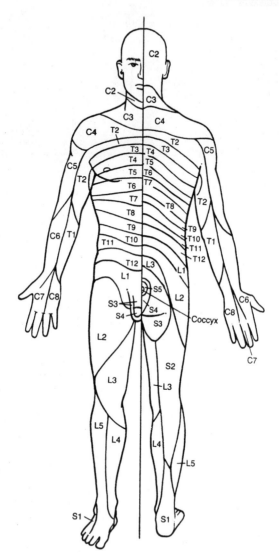

Skin areas innervated by spinal nerves (dermatomes).
From Monahan, F.D. et al. Nursing Care of Adults. Philadelphia; WB Saunders, 1994. p. 1456.

How to Do Breast Self-Examination

Do breast self-examination (BSE) every month. Become familiar with how your breasts usually look and feel. Do BSE to find any change from what is normal for you.

If you still menstruate, the best time to do BSE is 2 or 3 days after your period ends. These are the days when your breasts are least likely to be tender or swollen.

If you no longer menstruate, pick a certain day—such as the first day of each month—to remind yourself to do BSE.

If you are taking hormones, talk with your doctor about when to do BSE.

Here's what you should do to check for changes in your breasts.

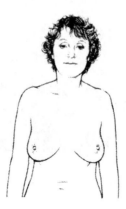

1. Stand in front of a mirror that is large enough for you to see your breasts clearly. Check each breast for anything unusual. Check the skin for puckering, dimpling, or scaliness. Look for a discharge from the nipples.

Do step 2 and 3 to check for any change in the shape or contour of your breasts. As you do these steps, you should feel your chest muscles tighten.

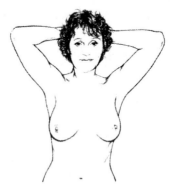

2. Watching closely in the mirror, clasp your hands behind your head and press your hands forward.

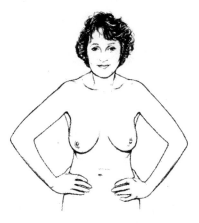

3. Next, press your hands firmly on your hips and bend slightly toward the mirror as you pull your shoulders and elbows forward.

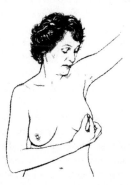

4. Gently squeeze each nipple and look for a discharge.

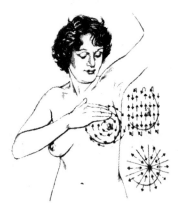

5. Raise one arm. Use the pads of the fingers of your other hand to check the breast and the surrounding area—firmly, carefully, and thoroughly. Some women like to use lotion or powder to help their fingers glide easily over the skin. Feel for any unusual lump or mass under the skin.

Feel the tissue by pressing your fingers in small, overlapping areas about the size of a dime. To be sure you cover your whole breast, take your time and follow a definite pattern, lines, circles, or wedges.

Some research suggests that many women do BSE more thoroughly when they use a pattern of up-and-down lines or strips. Other women feel more comfortable with another pattern. The important thing is to cover the whole breast and to pay special attention to the area between the breast and the underarm, including the underarm itself. Check the area above the breast, up to the collarbone and all the way over to your shoulder.

Lines: Start in the underarm area and move your fingers downward little by little until they are below the breast. Then move your fingers slightly toward the middle and slowly move back up. Go up and down until you cover the whole area.

Circles: Beginning at the outer edge of your breast, move your fingers slowly around the whole breast in a circle. Move around the breast in smaller and smaller circles, gradually working toward the nipple. Don't forget to check the underarm and upper chest areas, too.

Wedges: Starting at the outer edge of the breast, move your fingers toward the nipple and back to the edge. Check your whole breast, covering one small wedge-shaped section at a time. Be sure to check the underarm area and the upper chest.

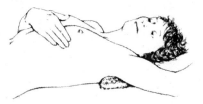

6. It's important to repeat step 5 while you are lying down. Lie flat on your back, with one arm over your head and a pillow or folded towel under the opposite shoulder. The position flattens the breast and makes it easier to check. Check each breast and the area around it very carefully using one of the patterns described above.

7. Some women repeat step 5 in the shower. Your fingers will glide easily over soapy skin, so you can concentrate on feeling for changes underneath.

If you notice a lump, a discharge, or any other change during the month—whether or not it is during BSE—contact your doctor.

Technique for breast self-examination. (Courtesy of the National Cancer Institute.)

Appendix 8
Testicular Self-Examination

The most common symptom of testicular cancer is a small pea-sized mass on the front or side of the testicle. Testicular cancer is highly curable, particularly when treated early in its development. Because a small mass can be felt on testicular self-examination (TSE) before any other symptoms develop, TSE allows early detection and treatment and increases the chances of cure.

TSE PROCEDURE

Perform TSE once a month after a warm bath or shower, because the heat relaxes the scrotal skin and makes it easier to feel anything unusual.

Stand naked in front of a mirror. Look for any swelling on the skin of the scrotum.

Examine each testicle gently with both hands. The index and middle fingers should be placed underneath the testicle while the thumbs are placed on the top. Roll the testicle gently between the thumbs and fingers. One testicle may be larger than the other.

Find the epididymis (a cordlike structure on the top and
  back of the testicle that stores and transports the sperm).
  Do not confuse the epididymis with an abnormal lump.
Feel for a small lump—about the size of pea—on the front
  or the side of the testicle. These lumps are usually painless (see Figure).
Contact the doctor immediately if a lump is found.

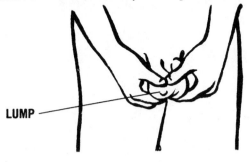

LUMP

*Adapted from National Cancer Institute. Testicular self-examination.
(National Institutes of Health Publication No. 92-2636.) Washington,
DC: U.S. Department of Health and Human Services, Public Health
Service, 1992.*

Appendix 9
Signs of Physical Abuse

Consider the possibility of physical abuse when a patient presents with:

a history of repeated accidents or trauma.

concealed or unexplained injuries.

an apparent discrepancy between the history of trauma and the type of injury incurred.

acute embarrassment over a seemingly non-embarrassing incident.

GERIATRIC CONSIDERATIONS

Consider the possibility of abuse of the elderly when the patient presents with:

signs of physical trauma such as fingerprint bruises on the upper arms, bruises on the inner thighs, or other unexplained injuries.

signs of neglect such as dirty, long nails; matted hair; thick corns and calluses; soiled clothing; body or mouth odor.

signs of psychological abuse such as reports of long periods of isolation.

PEDIATRIC CONSIDERATIONS

Abuse is suspected and/or diagnosed by identifying a combination of signs and symptoms. The only *single* symptom that validates sexual abuse is confirmed STD in an otherwise sexually inactive child. Possible signs of physical abuse in a child include:

Failure to thrive
Unexplained injuries
Injuries where the explanation does not fit the type of injury
Bruises in various stages of healing especially in areas other than those where children frequently bang themselves when playing
Multiple fractures
Cigarette burns
Burns on lower extremities, hands, and buttocks
Behavior and emotional problems
Poor school performance
Decreased attention span
Aggravated fears

Possible signs of sexual abuse in a child include:

Precocious sexual knowledge and/or play
Genital, throat, and/or anal STD's
Trauma to the genitalia
Behavior and emotional problems
Poor school performance
Aggravated fears
Decreased attention span

Clinical Note

Obtain an uncoached history from a child or adolescent in his/her own words.

From Monahan, F.D. et al. Nursing Care of Adults. Philadelphia; WB Saunders, 1994.

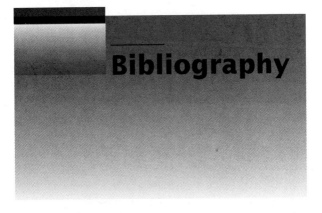

Bibliography

Ablon, GR and Rosen, T. Cutaneous signs of systemic disease: a guide to gleaning diagnostic clues from the skin. Consultant, 1994 Apr; 34(4): 495-9, 503-4, 506.

Adult screening for cancer detection: thyroid examination and function: seventh in a series of articles based on chapters exerpted from the Clinician's Handbook of Clinical Preventative Services, part of the Put Prevention into Practice Program from the US Public Health Service. Nurse Pract, 1995 May; 20(5): 64, 66-7.

Assessing Patients. Springhouse, Pa: Springhouse, 1996.

Balakas, K and Schappe, A. Procedures in home care. Well baby assessment. Home Healthcare Nurse, 1995 Sep-Oct; 13(5): 82-84.

Bates, B. A guide to physical examination and history taking 6th ed. Philadelphia: Lippincott, 1995.

Bynum, WF and Porter, R. (eds). Medicine and the five senses. New York: Cambridge University Press, 1993.

Cancer detection by physical examination: breast and pelvic organ examination. Nurs Pract, 1994 Oct; 19(10), 20-2, 24.

Caulker-Burnett, I. Primary care screening for substance abuse. Nurs Pract, 1994 Jun; 19(6): 42, 44-8.

Daniger, L. Clinical breast exam training and breast self exam teaching: a challenge to nurses. Minn Nurs Accent. 1994 Apr; 66(4): 6.

DeGowin, RL. DeGowin & DeGowin's diagnostic examination 6th ed. New York: McGraw-Hill, 1994.

Dienger, MJ and Llewellyn, J. Increasing compliance with breast self examination. Medsurg Nurs, 1995 Oct; 4(5): 359-366.

Fowlie, P and Forsyth, S. Examination of the newborn infant. Modern Midwife, 1995 Jan; 5(1): 15-8.

Freeborne, N. The functionally oriented assessment of the geriatric patient. Journal of the American Academy of Physician Assistants, 1994 Mar; 7(3): 158-67, 29A.

Greenberger, NJ. History taking and physical examination: essentials and clinical correlates. St. Louis: Mosby–Yearbook, 1993.

Kanski, KK. Clinical ophthalmology: a systematic approach 3rd ed. Boston: Butterworth-Heinemann, 1994.

Kelsher, KC. Primary care for women: environmental assessment of the home, community, and workplace. J Nurse Midwife, 1995 Mar-Apr; 40(2): 59-64, 88-96.

Misulis, KE. Neurologic localization and diagnosis. Boston: Butterworth-Heinemann, 1996.

Morrissey, J. Obtaining a "reasonably accurrate" health history. Plastic Surgical Nursing 1994 Spring; 14(1): 27-30.

Poncar, PJ. Who has time for a 'head-to-toe' assessment? Nursing, 1995 Mar; 25(3): 59.

Pressman, EK, Zeidman, SM, Summers L. Primary care for women: comprehensive assessment of the neurologic system. J Nurse Midwife, 1995 Mar-Apr; 40(2): 59-64, 163-171.

Seidel, HM, Ball, JW, Dains, JE, and Benedict, GW. Mosby's guide to physical examination, 3rd edition. St. Louis: Mosby–Yearbook, 1995.

Seymour, CA. Clinical clerking: a short introduction to clinical skills 2nd ed. New York: Cambridge University Press, 1994.

Silverman, ME and Hurst, JW. Clinical skills for adult primary care. Philadelphia: Lippincott-Raven, 1995.

Swartz, MH. Textbook of Physical Diagnosis. Philadelphia: WB Saunders, 1995.

Unti, SM. The critical first year of life: history, physical assessment, and general developmental assessment. Pediatr Clin North Am, 1994 Oct; 41(5): 859-873.

Vessey, JA. Primary care approaches. Developmental approaches in examining young children. Pediatr Nurs, 1995 Jan-Feb; 21(1): 53-6.

Weilitz, PB and Lueckenotte, A. Respiratory assessment of older adults: part II. Perspectives in respiratory nursing, 1995 May; 6(2): 1, 3-4.

Wilkins, RL, Krider, SJ, and Sheldon, RL. Clinical assessment in respiratory care. St. Louis: Mosby–Yearbook, 1995.

Willms, JL. Physical diagnosis: bedside evaluation of diagnosis and function. Baltimore: Williams & Wilkins, 1994.

Wilson, D. Assessing and managing the febrile child. Nurse Pract, 1995 Nov; 20(11 part 1): 59-60, 68-74.

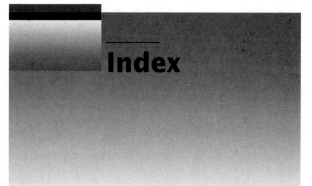

Index

Note: Page numbers in *italic* refer to illustrations; those followed by t refer to tables.